Dr Mike
AI

Dr Mike Smith is a spe
and a general practition
Officer of the Family
and their Honorary Medical Adviser 1975–90. He is an elected member of the FPA's National Executive Committee, a member of the Pet Health Council and a member of the advisory panel of the National Food Safety Advisory Centre. For many years he has been a 'resident' expert guest on BBC Radio 2's *Jimmy Young Show*, LBC's *Nightline* and the medical columnist/editor for *Woman's Own*. Between 1988 and 1990 he was the expert guest on SKY TV's *Sky by Day*. In April 1991 he was voted the TV and Radio Doctors' 'Expert's Expert' in the *Observer* magazine's series.

As well as the Postbag series, he is also the author of *Birth Control, How to Save Your Child's Life, A New Dictionary of Symptoms, Dr Mike Smith's Handbook of Over-the-Counter Medicines, Dr Mike Smith's Handbook of Prescription Medicines* and *Dr Mike Smith's First Aid Handbook* (to be published May 1994).

DR MIKE SMITH'S
POSTBAG

ALLERGIES

WITH SHARRON KERR

KYLE CATHIE LIMITED

First published in Great Britain in 1994 by
Kyle Cathie Limited
7/8 Hatherley Street, London SW1P 2QT

ISBN 1 85626 124 7

A Cataloguing in Publication record for this title is
available from the British Library.

Typeset by Heronwood Press, Medstead, Hampshire
Printed in Great Britain by Cox and Wyman Ltd, Reading

CONTENTS

INTRODUCTION

I am often asked just how common allergies are. Are they on the increase or is it just that we hear more about them these days? As we are getting more health-conscious, do we now examine the finer details of our well-being much more? Or are we just becoming a nation of hypochondriacs, as one letter writer put it!

People seem to be interested in knowing more about allergies. I don't base that just on the number of letters I receive in my postbag asking about them, but on the extensive column inches given to all manner of allergies from the unusual to the extreme and fatal. There have even been newspaper reports of a child being allergic to solid food, who survives on special milk and Fox's Glacier Mints. Other reports include the story of a pupil who suffered headaches and stomach problems throughout his A-level year at school after eating school meals containing flour. He turned out to have a severe allergy to wheat protein and won £3000 compensation. The *British Medical Journal* recounted the story of a man in his thirties who had an acute reaction to a mango – a fruit he'd eaten for the first time – resulting in a widespread rash, puffy eyes, red face and difficulty breathing. But I have to add this is very unusual.

More recent and even more serious newspaper reports have told of the extremely rare but fatal consequences of unsuspectingly eating food containing nuts to which one is allergic. Within two hours of biting a nut in an Indian take-away meal, one woman died from acute anaphylaxis, an allergic reaction which can cause victims to choke to death (see page 71). Another woman died a few hours after eating a lemon meringue pie which had finely crushed peanuts sprinkled on top, while a schoolgirl died after eating a peanut-flavoured biscuit. Such incidents have added further emphasis to the need for better food labelling.

In answer to questions as to whether or not we are developing more allergies, some figures do suggest that over the last ten years more people are consulting their GP about these problems, in particular hay fever and asthma. Some experts believe that because, as a nation, we are becoming healthier, we are also becoming prone to allergic reactions from substances that might not have affected us before. It is suggested that as the infectious diseases are brought under control in the developed world, our immune system then starts to over-react to these substances, coming to identify them as harmful invaders, and treating them as if they were germs.

Another theory is that as the air we breathe becomes more polluted through industry and the motor car, air pollutants may make the lungs more vulnerable to allergens such as pollens and viruses. According to the National Asthma Campaign, exhaust fumes, one of the main pollutants, have increased by 75 per cent since 1980. The situation isn't likely to improve that much either because although some cars have catalytic converters, many older cars do not, coupled with the fact that traffic volume could easily more than double within the next thirty years.

The popular media have even carried reports about sufferers who were supposedly allergic to the twentieth century! They were said to be reacting in a many-symptom way to the various irritants that our modern way of life and manufacturing processes put into our environment, both intentionally, as with detergents, and unintentionally, as with pollutants. It was claimed that they had to live in a totally controlled environment in order to be free of the symptoms. However I have yet to be convinced that this was the case.

This is not to say that there aren't processes which will cause accepted allergies, for example, the hardening of some soft metals and plastics with nickel. Nickel, when worn next to the skin, can sensitise the wearer to it, causing both a local reaction – rash – as well as an all-over-the-body reaction, either a rash or other symptoms such as the swelling of oedema. An allergy to cement is another common problem.

But there have been so many unsubstantiated claims about allergies that objective observers require a more measurable standard of proof before they are convinced that an allergy is the cause of a problem. Most doctors and scientists therefore tend to keep their distance and, as a result, are often criticised for being too cynical.

I'm keeping my options open!

WHAT IS AN ALLERGY?

An allergy is the result of the body's defence mechanism going into top gear. An allergen is any substance in the environment which when taken into the body may cause it to become hypersensitive. The body can over-react when harmless substances, such as pollen in the air or pet hairs, are 'viewed' by the body's defence system (antibodies) as foreign. The antibodies in the sufferer's blood – produced to protect us from germs – may then react to the allergen, releasing powerful chemicals which cause the symptoms of the allergy, for example a skin rash, excessive secretions in the nose or eyes, or spasm of the bronchial muscles (asthma). (Tests show that those prone to an allergy tend to have a much higher concentration of one particular type of antibody in their blood known as immunoglobulin E – IgE for short.)

The antibodies attack our mast cells (large cells found in the skin, nose, lungs and intestines), releasing the chemical histamine and at least seven other substances which cause the tiny blood vessels (capillaries) to dilate and their walls to leak. Of course, when an infection is the cause this is good for the body as the dilated blood vessels bring in more blood cells to deal with the invaders and the secretion dilutes the infectious agent and helps wash it out of the nose.

An allergic reaction can take many guises. Sufferers can experience difficulties in breathing as in an asthma attack, bouts of constant sneezing, a runny nose, itchy eyes, swelling of the eyes, lips or other parts of the body, dizziness, an upset stomach, diarrhoea, migraine, eczema, urticaria and difficulties with the cardio-vascular system, causing acute shock and, if it's not treated quickly, cardiac failure.

WHAT CAUSES AN ALLERGY?

I've lost count of the number of questions I've received about allergies, probably because they affect around a quarter of us at some time in our lives; certainly the subject does arouse quite a lot of interest, and anxiety. One of the most common worries is whether or not allergies run in families. The answer is yes. Evidence seems to suggest that allergies do have some connection with heredity – it's all in the genes. If both your parents suffer from an allergy there is a 60 per cent likelihood that you will too. Other estimates suggest the risk could be as high as seven out of ten. If only one of your parents has allergies the risk is obviously less and goes down to a 30–50 per cent chance. Although bear in mind that it's not the actual allergy itself that you are likely to inherit, but the susceptibility to allergic reactions because you'll probably develop the IgE antibody. Consequently, this makes you susceptible to any allergy, not necessarily a specific one.

As well as being born with an inherited tendency are there any other things that could spark off an allergy? Some research suggests that in childhood a virus such as the common cold or an episode of influenza could trigger off an allergy, but generally only when both parents have the tendency to allergic reactions.

Does stress play a role in allergy? It's too easy to say that it does, because the automatic response to any allergy that gets worse while a sufferer is going through a period of pressure is to blame the stress – even when there is no evidence that this is the cause. In fact, during periods of stress the body actually secretes more adrenaline and natural steroids, both of which, as medicines, can be used to *treat* allergies. My opinion is that stress doesn't play a major part in a true allergy – it just looks as though it does because stress is so common that it is often present when the allergy gets worse.

How long is an allergic reaction likely to last? This one is very difficult to answer as each individual's response is different. Equally, the length of time taken for an allergy to develop varies from person to person. While some people only have to be exposed to something once to produce an allergic reaction – for example, the first time you eat a prawn – others will find that sensitisation to, say, dogs may take many months or even years of exposure.

This book is not intended for self-diagnosis – its purpose is to inform. If you think you have an allergy then do discuss the problem with your GP.

Here I will discuss the most common types of allergy, including case studies of many sufferers to highlight the problems experienced. I hope their experiences will 'comfort' similar sufferers and promote understanding in those who are lucky enough not to have trouble with allergies. I also discuss some allergy-related questions that I'm often asked, and in later chapters I talk about, and offer advice on, treatment and the best ways to cope.

1: HAY FEVER

To the many millions of British people who suffer from hay fever, the green countryside poses a threat instead of an idyll. When the grasses start to disperse their millions of microscopical pollen grains those sufferers begin sneezing, have a runny, bunged-up nose and irritated red and watery eyes. There's a fair chance too that they will develop a wheezy chest, a sore throat, lethargy and malaise and even itching ears, similar in fact to a full-blown infection of the lining membrane of the upper respiratory tract.

Pollen in the hypersensitive hay fever sufferer produces similar tissue responses and bodily feelings to invasion and infection by the common germ allergens. We've all had a streaming cold, and therefore know what this can mean symptomatically. Pollens can also trigger symptoms of asthma, such as coughing, chestiness and wheeziness.

Hay fever is an allergic reaction which occurs in people who are particularly sensitive to pollen or spores released into the air by trees, grasses or moulds. The problem's medical name is seasonal allergic rhinitis, or seasonal allergic rhino conjunctivitis, and it is one of the most common allergies known. And it's an allergy that's on the increase, probably due to increasing pollution. It's difficult to pinpoint exactly how common it is or how many people suffer from it because for some it is more of a debilitating problem than a disabling one. Many people, I know, don't even bother to visit their GP about it, preferring instead to buy a remedy from the pharmacist. Certainly the over-the-counter market for anti-allergy products (the antihistamines) runs into millions of pound each year. However it is estimated that in the UK one person in ten suffers, while other figures suggest it's even higher and could affect as many as one in five. As a consequence it's estimated that four million working days are lost during June and July alone through hay fever.

All sections of the population are possible sufferers, but men are slightly more at risk than women. I've even read that studies have suggested if a baby is born during the pollen season, he or she is more likely to develop hay fever in later life! Hay fever peaks in the early teens (although it's common between the ages of ten and forty) and often runs in the family. It may adversely affect holidays and school work, particularly exams that have an importance for one's future career. Later in the teens, twenties and thirties, work is affected too. Happily, the condition does tend to get better with age.

Hay fever strictly refers to an allergy to grass pollen, but the term is often used to cover allergies to the pollen from plants, shrubs and trees. The symptoms experienced are due not to the pollen itself, but to the body's *reaction* to it. During an attack, catechol amines (around twenty different chemicals, including histamine) are released from the mast cells in the tissues. These amines attract the white blood cells (platelets), which are part of the body's defence mechanism to fight infection and which are known to be associated with inflammation. The ones mainly attracted are the eosinophils – so called because they can be stained with eosin to stand out from the others when viewed under a microscope.

The concentration of these cells sets up a damaging inflammatory reaction similar to that which would deal with a dangerous germ invasion. In the case of hay fever, however, the sufferer has to put up with the 'battle' which was not necessary in the first place for the pollen would not otherwise have caused harm.

The eyes water in an effort to wash away the pollen and the runing nose and sneezing help to eject the 'invader'. Virtually all sufferers get nasal symptoms, eight out of ten eye symptoms and as many as six out of ten 'pollen' wheezing as well. Of this latter group, the misery of the symptoms can, rarely, be overshadowed by the more serious acute asthmatic attack requiring hospital treatment for its relief.

Pollens released in spring are usually from trees and can produce the same symptoms as grass pollen, while in the summer flowers, grass or weed pollens are released. June and July are the worst months for the grass pollens, but lawn-mowing in the preceding weeks may bring on the symptoms earlier, ruining the best summer months for many people. In the autumn symptoms are usually caused by pollen from autumn-flowering plants and the spores of some fungi.

Hay fever sufferers are most at risk between May and September, when the 'pollen count' (the level of pollen in the air) is at its highest. Listen to the pollen count forecasts broadcast daily on television and local radio or check the weather reports in the newspaper (a count of fifty grains per cubic metre is enough to set most sufferers sneezing). The pollen count will be high on warm, dry days, when pollen is released, and particularly so when it is windy because the spores released from grasses and trees are carried upwards by warm air.

Symptoms are often more severe in the morning when pollen is released. They are carried higher into the air as the temperature rises, so symptoms can become worse again in the evening as the temperature drops and the pollen grains drift back down. The symptoms will also tend to be worse in those years when the weather is colder or wetter than usual. Dry pollen is lighter than air and can readily disperse on warm air currents. But when it is wet the pollen grains are more likely to clump together, and without the help from the warm air as it rises they are less able to lift off.

Diagnosis is usually straightforward. The nature of the symptoms, the time of year, physical examination and occasionally a blood test will all help. For the first time sufferer from a non-suffering family, the age old rhetoric will usually be posed: 'It can't be hay fever, Doc. I've never had it before.'

With as many as one in six teenagers suffering from hay fever, the allergy is a nuisance and extra element of stress for those sitting exams. I sometimes wonder how many examiners understand what a handicap it can be for some youngsters. So think ahead. If you or a member of your family has suffered in the past and is planning to take examinations in the pollen season you should make sure your doctor has been consulted and the best form of treatment decided upon. And make sure this treatment is taken as soon as practicably possible.

Joy, a thirty-four-year-old computer analyst, who is also sensitive to cats, finds that although she developed hay fever as a teenager it still gives her a runny nose and itchy eyes. She also experiences slight itching in her throat and lots of sneezing which makes driving difficult when she's wearing her contact lenses because her vision can become blurred.

Fortunately, as she works full-time and the building has an efficient air-conditioning system, her symptoms are minimised these days, which wasn't the case when she was taking her O-levels.

At work we have air-conditioning which is great. I can tell the difference as soon as I come out at night and the pollen begins to affect me again.

It's more of a problem at weekends. I don't like too many antihistamines; I find they don't always work anyway so I try not to take them throughout the day and night. At weekends if I know we are going out in the evening I save the dosage for mid-afternoon so it's most likely to work for that particular evening.

Like many hay fever sufferers, especially those who have experienced the allergy each summer for many years, Joy prefers to try to ignore it as much as she can.

I do tend to soldier on. But one thing really makes me bad and that's the smell of nettles. If we go for a walk in the evening along the canal bank, which we do if we are going to the pub in the summer, and we have a stroll before or after the drink, that really tends to set my hay fever off. I don't let hay fever affect my life so I don't tend to avoid things but by just carrying on it can certainly makes things more uncomfortable at times.

For Joy, her worst experiences with hay fever happened while she was at school.

It really started when I was in my teens around about the age of fourteen. It was at the same time as my cat allergy started – I haven't always been allergic to cats. When I was taking my O-levels it was so bad that it used to give me nose bleeds. I'd be in an exam and I'd have a nose bleed. It was quite distressing, especially when my O-levels results were riding on my performance. I had a friend who got it at the same time as me. And her nose bleeds were even worse. She had them all the time, where I would have a couple a week. But during one exam it was so bad I had to leave the room and then come back later and was allowed a little more time to complete the paper.

Nose bleeds are caused because the reaction to pollen is inflammatory in nature. This means that the affected areas are swollen and the blood vessels more 'breakable'. Consequently, nose bleeds are more likely to occur, especially in someone susceptible to them. Nose bleeds can usually be quickly stopped by squeezing shut the front, soft part of the nose between the thumb and first finger and breathing through the mouth for a few moments. If you're in the exam room it's worth drawing it to the attention of the examiner, like Joy did, and asking for extra time to compensate.

Other sufferers may want to ignore their hay fever and soldier on regardless, but the severity of their symptoms often prevents them from even attempting this strategy. Terry, a thirty-seven-year-old decorator, has put up with some dreadful summers because of his hay fever.

Thankfully I don't get it as bad as I used to. I remember reading once that hay fever is probably more common in cities and towns than in the countryside. At first I was surprised to learn that. But when I think about it, I was born and brought up in West London and I certainly knew a lot of people who suffered, some of them even worse than me.

I must have developed hay fever when I was about ten. I remember that one of my best friends had it and I was really jealous! You know how it is: when you're that age you want what your mates have got. What a thing to wish on yourself!

I didn't have it when I was younger because when they used to mow the grass outside our block of flats the gardeners would leave it in big piles. My friends and I used to roll around in the piles of mown grass with no effect at all.

One year I just started sneezing and my nose began to stream. It was like having a cold, but I think hay fever is much worse than a cold because for three months or so there's no respite from it. I remember coming home from school and having to lie on the bed with a damp flannel on my face. That was the only way I could get any relief.

I have a photo of myself on holiday in the Isle of Wight when I was about sixteen and my hay fever was so bad my eyes had swollen up. Just looking at that photo makes me shudder even now and it reminds me of how I was feeling that day. I was completely bunged up and felt awful.

For Terry getting through the day was bad enough, but dealing with his hay fever at night was often even worse.

It's easier to forget what a pain hay fever is during the day when you are busy. Although having said that, it was horrendous when I worked for a firm, rather than being self-employed, and I had to turn up no matter what. My job as a decorator inevitably involved rubbing down walls and creating more dust to irritate my already inflamed nose and eyes. I don't know how I coped some days but I just got on with it. Since I've been self-employed I just stay at home with the windows shut if I have a very bad day.

I used to wipe my nose so much I'd get sores around my nose and on my top lip. My nose would run all night as well and the moisture streaming out would irritate me and wake me up. I used to get so fed up of waking just to wipe my nose. In the end I used to get a great big dollop of Vaseline and smooth it all around my nose. Then I would lie on my side and put a towel under my nose. That way I could let my nose run into the towel and it wouldn't wake me up. I'd wake in the morning and the towel would be soaked. My nose really did run like a tap. I also used to wake feeling really dehydrated.

I know that pollen is supposed to be given out by grass in the morning and that it rises as the day goes on and that as night falls so does the pollen. That does make you feel worse but the other thing that would make it seem worse at night, like any illness, is that when things are still and quiet it's hard to relax and forget about what's troubling you.

Hay fever has meant that Terry often can't go out as much as he wants, although he tries not to let it rule his life. But, as he says, that's difficult when on top of all the usual symptoms, he has violent sneezing fits.

I could have a fit of a dozen or even more sneezes. I would sneeze really loudly and violently. Sometimes it seemed as if I was never going to stop. That used to be so exhausting.

Then one of my sneezing attacks forced me to have a week off work when I really hurt my back. I was bending down at work – I had been sneezing all day – when I felt a sneeze coming on. I let it go while I was crouched over. By doing that I yanked a muscle in my back. So my advice to other sufferers is, if you are going to sneeze make sure you stand up first!

As summer coincides with so many sufferers' annual holiday, it can spoil that much-awaited break. Terry was no exception. His hay fever almost ruined a four-month tour when he drove around Europe with friends in a camper van.

I went on a long summer holiday and I'd been looking forward to it for ages but I think it must have been my worst hay fever season ever. My friends only told me years later that I drove them completely mad because of my heavy breathing and constant sniffing at night. When they were all trying to sleep I was blowing my nose and sneezing.

It totally spoilt the first part of my holiday. I remember we stopped in Paris for a few days. I was so bad I was doubling the dose of antihistamines and they had no effect at all. That also makes me shudder even now just thinking about how awful I felt. We spent three days driving down to the South of France and by the time I got to the coast I just wanted to go home. Sometimes the pink membrane at the corner of my eye would swell up and at its worst in France it covered about a third of my eye.

I tried to take measures to help myself but nothing much helped. I did wear dark glasses but only because no one can see your dark puffed-up eyes; they didn't help much in any other way even though my doctor reckoned they might help keep pollen away from my eyes. I used to try all the antihistamines on the market. All of a sudden one would work for a few days then it would be hopeless so I'd go out and buy another brand.

As well as holidays another thing that was a problem for me was driving in May, June and July and not being able to have the car windows open. It was either drive home from work sneezing or drive home sweating. I didn't know which was worse, they were both so uncomfortable. At least now some new cars have pollen filters. What a breakthrough.

It's only fellow sufferers who know how horrible hay fever can be. The thing that used to drive me mad was when people would tell me that it was all in the mind!

Hay fever does often subside as the sufferer gets older. Among the many forms in which the body's chemistry reacts to an allergy – known as allergic pathways – there is one process by which desensitisation occurs and the body becomes less sensitive. It tends to do this with hay fever and, fortunately for Terry, seems to be happening in his case.

I have been better for the past few years. I guess it must be for the last five or six years. I have a lot more summer holidays early on in the season. I try to go away for two weeks in May to Ibiza. As that has a fairly arid landscape it means I can have a trouble-free holiday. And somehow getting away from London early in the summer helped. It set me up for the rest of summer – if I didn't get 'stung' at the beginning of the season the rest of the pollen season wasn't so bad for me. I also think the medication available is better now and Beconase has helped me a lot in recent years. So I believe that in my case a combination of getting older and the improved treatment now available has meant that hay fever is no longer the problem it used to be.

This has meant a great deal to me because hay fever when you get it as badly as I have done spoils the best part of the summer – May and June, when everything is so fresh and you've looked forward to it all winter.

2: PERENNIAL RHINITIS

Having a cold once or twice a year, as most of us do, is bad enough – imagine what it would be like to have cold-like symptoms all year round. Probably about one person in ten – young or old – suffers in this way.

Rhinitis is simply an inflammation of the mucous membrane lining the nose and there are many possible causes. Seasonal rhinitis (see Hay Fever, pages 7–15) occurs as an allergic reaction to pollens and other allergens around at a particular time of year – in between the symptoms disappear and the sufferer tends to forget all about it, until the next spring and summer. In the case of perennial rhinitis, however, the nose remains inflamed and the unpleasant symptoms – which may include a constantly blocked or runny nose, itchy eyes and frequent sneezing – persist. The sense of taste and smell can also be affected and the sufferer often feels generally 'under the weather'. If he or she experiences these symptoms for more than one hour in twenty-four on most days of the year, a diagnosis of perennial rhinitis can be made. Children who suffer from perennial rhinitis typically develop a 'nose crease' from constantly rubbing their itchy nose upwards. Nose bleeds are also quite common and dark circles under the eyes may be another sign.

In a few cases these continuing symptoms will be due to a physical obstruction in the nose, such as polyps. Sometimes they will be a reaction to certain drugs, to changes in hormone levels – during pregnancy and at the menopause, for instance – or to changes in temperature or humidity. Irritating conditions at work, such as smoke or fumes, can also be responsible. Most often, however, symptoms are due to an allergy, for example, to animal fur and hair or to house-dust mites, invisible to the naked eye, which exist in their millions in the furnishings, floors and bedding of even the cleanest home.

Mike, a thirty-eight-year-old marketing executive, had suffered from perennial rhinitis for many years before it was diagnosed. He'd always thought he suffered constantly from chills and colds, because he never seemed to be without a runny nose. He knew too that he was allergic to cats and dogs (see page 32), but it was only when he saw an ear, nose and throat specialist (about a recurrent problem with tonsillitis) that he discovered he'd been suffering from perennial rhinitis as well.

The specialist advised me to have my tonsils taken out because I kept getting bouts of tonsillitis. I also had my sinuses washed out at the same time because I suffered a lot with sinus headaches as well. When he had examined me the specialist told me that I had a deviated septum which I'd already been told when I was a child. But to my surprise he told me that most of the problem with my sinuses and my constant 'colds' was due to perennial rhinitis and that this was most likely being caused by an allergy to the house-dust mite.

In a way I was relieved to be told this because I'd thought there was something wrong with me. It didn't seem healthy to be constantly full of cold. I used to spend days feeling not quite right, under the weather but not really knowing why. I had so often bought decongestant sprays to try to get rid of the bunged up feelings and in the hope of drying up my runny nose, but I realised then that I had probably done more harm than good. The doctor explained to me that using these sprays too much can sometimes make matters worse by causing a rebound congestion. At least now I knew that there were some things I could do to help alleviate the situation. I had no idea that house-dust mites could be the cause of so many uncomfortable symptoms.

HOUSE-DUST MITES

If you think you'll be able to learn more about house-dust mites without scratching then do read on! The house-dust mite is a microscopic eight-legged 'beast' which lives – and thrives – on the dead skin cells that we shed constantly, particularly in bed. It's thought that we each shed approximately four pounds of these dead skin cells each year, so you can see the house-dust mite's diet is in plentiful supply.

Each of these millions of mites produces twenty to forty faecal pellets a day – not a pretty thought! Fortunately, most of us co-exist quite happily with the mites, but the pellets are the trigger that provokes the allergic response and symptoms of perennial rhinitis in the susceptible. The faeces remain allergenic even after the mite that produced them has died, at the end of its three- to four-month lifespan.

The trouble is caused by a digestive enzyme in these faeces, compounded by the fact that the faecal particles break down into very small pieces which are roughly the size of a grain of pollen. And just like pollen they are easily borne into the air, which is how they are inhaled or come into contact with skin. When inhaled the body's reaction, in those who are susceptible, is to treat the enzyme as an allergen and provoke an allergic reaction.

These mites are now thought to play a major role in allergies such as asthma, allergic rhinitis and eczema. One study carried out in the late 1980s showed that asthmatic patients demonstrated up to a 40 per cent reduction in both asthma attacks and symptoms when they were moved to an environment which was mite-free. A later study carried out in Denmark showed that if a person had high levels of house-dust mites in their homes they were five times more likely to suffer from eczema than those who lived in environments low in the mites.

House-dust mites continue to thrive because modern conditions provide them with perfect breeding grounds. They love the warmth of our centrally heated homes and the humidity too, which is not only provided by central heating but also by double glazing and house insulation. All these heat conservation measures mean that our homes are less draughty than they used to be, making them warmer and cosier for the mite. Some experts believe that as the fashion for fitted carpets has spread so have attacks of allergic asthma. Soft furnishings, too, provide an ideal environment with an average home giving plenty of choice – lots of full curtains, frilly blinds and cosy, comfy sofas. Many of us sleep on mattresses which are several years old. Just think how much skin and perspiration they must have absorbed in that time given that we spend an average of eight hours a night in bed.

One letter writer told me that a couple of years ago her mother started sneezing a lot, particularly in the morning. She'd read that the cause was likely to be an allergy to the house-dust mite in bedding, so had got rid of her feather pillows and replaced them with foam ones. But this didn't seem to help much. She wanted to know if I could suggest other steps she could take.

A regular early morning bout of sneezing, puffy eyes or itching can certainly often be caused by an individual's allergy to the house-dust mite. But so far the correspondent's mother had changed only her pillows and perhaps needed to do more. For example, her mattress should be thoroughly vacuumed and her duvets or blankets taken to the dry cleaners. And she should consider having the bedroom carpets and curtains steam-cleaned, too. As we shed most of our microscopically small skin flakes in the bedroom, it's most important that we remove all the dust traps, as well as the dust.

Sometimes feathers can provoke an allergic response in the vulnerable. Again this is probably due to the dust mite and to the 'dander' – the microscopical particles of feather – that can filter through the pillow case. Dust can more readily collect in feather than foam pillows, carrying the mites and their droppings with it. Covers which can be 'wet wiped' but which also allow air in and out of the pillow (so that they are not sweaty to lie on) are now available (see page 83). These act like a filter, keeping the dander and the dust mites inside.

Lynne, a twenty-two-year-old trainee accountant, had no idea feather pillows could affect her breathing or sinuses until she stayed overnight at a friend's house.

> I didn't sleep very well at all that night. After a while I found it quite difficult to breathe. My chest began to feel very tight. In the morning I felt very dry and chesty and quite groggy. It seemed to have affected my sinuses and I felt totally blocked up. I have noticed it several times since and it's always when I stay elsewhere and sleep with feather pillows. So naturally I now avoid them wherever I can.

House-dust as well as the mites themselves can cause problems for other allergy-prone individuals. For Tom, a forty-six-year-old builder, it was an unfortunate allergy for someone whose main occupational pastime was creating clouds of it!

> The symptoms I used to get when exposed to house-dust were just like the symptoms I used to have when I suffered from hay fever as an adolescent. Hay fever had made school pretty grim at times. Compared with other people at school who didn't seem to be that bad, I was particularly sensitive. Now, at work, I found that I'd sneeze time after time after time. I'd have real bouts of it.
>
> I remember in particular the hot summer of 1976. I was working in an old cottage in Devon. I was pulling up floorboards which caused a terrific amount of dust. I suppose the natural humidity keeps a lot of the dust down, but in this instance the house was old, the boards very dry and the air was also very dry. I was pulling up old carpets as well as lifting floorboards.
>
> Together with the dust and the dryness of the air, I was in an awful state. I couldn't stop sneezing, my eyes were watering so much they began to puff up, my nose was streaming. I had a sore throat. The only respite from it was to wash my face and eyes with cold water. The other respite was to get away from the house and to have a long walk by the river which helped ease my symptoms.

But staying in this house overnight meant that I would wake in the morning with breathing difficulties. It was terrible. Another time I was working in a two-hundred-year-old house and I had to pull down a ceiling.

Being a builder it did cause problems for me; once you start hammering on floorboards you create all sorts of dust or even just moving furniture around. At times it made it almost impossible for me to carry on with my job because of all my coughing, sneezing and streaming eyes and nose – as anyone who has suffered from such an allergy will understand.

When I was younger I used to think I was allergic to sex! Whenever I had sex I used to sneeze violently afterwards. I couldn't understand it. I realise now, putting two and two together, that it was all the thrashing around in sheets, and because of all the house-dust mites you can get in mattresses.

I can't even tolerate a duvet being shaken to make the bed – I haven't shaken a duvet for years. Fluffing up pillows and cushions has the same effect. My wife would try her best to keep the house-dust mite levels down. But any housework, dusting or hoovering had to be done early in the day. Hoovering would irritate my nose too.

With age my symptoms seemed to have subsided. My problem with house-dust must have lasted about twenty years. Now I seem to be developing another problem, although it's not that bad and only lasts for a week or two each year. Since we have moved out of London and are living in more of a country area and we have a much bigger garden, I think I am developing allergic reactions not to grass but to fungus spores. There are lots of different fungi in our garden. I've noticed that in the late autumn I get all my old hay fever symptoms again.

3: ASTHMA

Anyone who doesn't know much about asthma may find it surprising that this problem can be allergy-related. In fact, one of the most common causes of asthma is allergy, the most usual allergens being pollens, house-dust mites, feathers and animals. Also many people are not aware just how widespread asthma is. It's thought to affect around three million people in the UK, a figure which includes more than a quarter of a million schoolchildren. One letter I received expressed surprise that when the writer's nine-year-old asthma-suffering son went on a school trip for the weekend, five other children in the group had to take their inhalers.

Asthma affects about one child in ten, although some experts believe it could even be more than that. It is an inflammatory condition that causes a swelling and constriction of the lining membrane of the breathing tubes. At the same time the very small muscles in these tubes contract, narrowing them further. It produces a recurrent cough, tightness of the chest or a wheeze – or all three – causing difficulty breathing.

Asthma can run in families but that doesn't mean to say if you have asthma that any child of yours will automatically develop it. The condition is often contracted quite young, although it generally fades away with the onset of puberty. Growing up probably helps because as the sufferer gets older, the main airways grow, which makes the air-flow easier.

In Britain, about 2000 people a year die, and more end up brain-damaged, as a result of a serious asthma attack. One of the worrying statistics is that it is the only treatable condition in the Western world which is on the increase.

According to the British Allergy Foundation, allergic asthma is five times more common in Australia than in Britain and twenty times more common in Britain than in China or Hong Kong. I can only guess as to why this should be so, but it is likely to be due to the differences in temperature between the countries – higher temperatures will increase the dispersal of pollen, while humidity will reduce it. In these countries the types of plants will differ too – for example, there may be fewer plants that rely on airborne pollen transport. Altitude may also have an effect: the higher land is dryer and so more condusive to pollen, the lower (especially Hong Kong at sea level) more humid and so less favourable to pollen dispersal. Pollution can also increase the incidence of asthma attacks. Also the body types of the people – Oriental Chinese compared with Caucasian Australians and British – are likely to provoke different asthmatic responses.

Asthma isn't always caused by an allergy, however. It can be due, for example, to an overreaction of the lung-lining tissues to cold temperatures or to exercise. Chest infections can also trigger asthma. In someone who already has the problem, worry and anxiety and pressure at home or at work can make it worse. Asthma is often more than a physical condition, it can be a social one as well, with attacks induced by emotion – simple things like laughter or excitement can even bring on the symptoms.

But for many asthmatics the cause remains a mystery – it's just something they have to live with. Fortunately, though, most people can learn to control their asthma by taking the correct medication and by learning not to panic when they feel an attack coming on.

Kinaird, a sixty-five-year-old pensioner, tries to lead as normal a life as possible with the help of asthma medicines and by avoiding the trigger factors he knows will provoke an attack.

Avoiding all the triggers cuts down on my attacks of asthma and makes me feel that I have an element of control over my life, although it is difficult to avoid them all the time. I find that I cannot let a day go by without considering what I could be allergic to or trying to avoid that trigger. And even with being so careful I can still be caught out now and again. I can never go anywhere with the definite guarantee that I won't have an attack.

A couple of years ago I had a really bad asthma attack when my son-in-law bought a brand-new car. We went out for a drive but after only about five minutes the strong, 'new' smell began to affect my breathing. Whenever you buy something new there always seems to be a certain smell around it. I can't pinpoint exactly what it was about this particular smell, whether it was the vinyl or the new carpets in the car, or even the upholstery. All I do know is that it was one of the worst asthma attacks I have ever had. It began with my nose feeling irritated and I was then unable to breathe through it. I tried to cover my nose with a handkerchief to try to blot out the smell of the car.

My chest became tight not long after. It's as if there are doors inside your chest which are banging shut. You really do feel your airways closing down. It's extremely frightening. We had to turn around and come home as quickly as we could. By the time I reached home my breathing was becoming so difficult we had to send for the doctor. When he arrived he couldn't get into his bag quick enough to get what he needed to give me a life-saving injection. I'm quite sure if he hadn't given me an injection that particular attack was so bad I would have died.

Kinaird believes that learning to keep calm during an attack does help, as does sitting up straight. But sometimes keeping calm is easier said than done.

It's very easy for someone who has never experienced an asthma attack to tell you to keep calm. I know some asthma sufferers who describe an attack as if there was a heavy weight on their chest or as if they are being strangled. But after an asthma attack, you realise that it must be a sensation that's the nearest thing to being buried alive. You're conscious of the fact that you are alive but at the same time you feel as if you are being suffocated and you can't do anything about it.

The only thing you can do is sit up straight and not move. By sitting still you're not exerting yourself or putting any pressure on yourself. Moving makes things even worse and makes it even more difficult to breathe. You do reach the stage sometimes when you can hardly breathe at all and then it's difficult to keep calm and to try not to panic.

Without his asthma medicines, Kinaird believes his life would be virtually non-existent.

I rely on medications to cope with my asthma. I take Becloforte morning and night. If I didn't take it it would make me short of breath most of the time. When I suddenly feel short of breath, I take Ventolin. I also take it when I know I'm going to exert myself – if I'm going for a long walk or if I do any small DIY job around the house. I can't go anywhere without having medication by my side. I carry Ventolin in my pocket wherever I go. That gives me the confidence to try to get on with my life.

I've suffered with asthma for about eight years and over the years I have worked out many of my trigger factors. I do my best to avoid them whenever I can. Dogs and cats are trigger factors. Just the smell of dogs affects me. If I go into a house where there's a dog, even if the dog isn't around but there is a doggy smell to the house, my chest goes tight and I have to leave immediately.

All sorts of dust and wood smoke do it. If someone has a log fire I can't get too near it. New carpets bother me. I suppose because they give off lots of fluff and tiny fibres of wool for a few weeks. Flowers and plants are definite triggers. I've managed to work out exactly which ones. Geraniums and lupins are very bad for me. My daughter has lots of potted geraniums in her kitchen. When I am coming to stay she makes sure she removes them about a week before the visit. Tomato plants are another trigger. I do like growing tomatoes so I usually wear a mask and gloves when I'm dealing with them. I also make sure I keep them outside as soon as I can rather than in the garden shed.

Freshly cut grass is another thing that makes me wheeze. So my wife always has to mow our lawn. Lilac trees really affect me badly. I can't go anywhere near them. We had one in the garden which I loved but sadly it had to go and we cut it down.

I can't have any house plants at all. They seem to irritate me as well. One of my doctors said he was fed up of telling his patients that they needed to get rid of their house plants because they are one of the worst things people with chest problems can keep.

Central heating is another trigger, especially when the air becomes too warm and dusty. Gas fires and electric fires affect me – although electric ones are slightly better than gas ones.

House dust mites – I can't have feather pillows and duvets. I even take my own pillows with me wherever I go. Anywhere where dust is being created is a no-go area for me. My wife always has to do the vacuuming. If I have to do it then I wear a mask.

Car fumes – we've recently moved house to a much quieter street much higher up a hill because the fumes can trigger an attack. If I am walking down a street and the traffic is moving slowly I notice it very quickly. My breathing is affected very easily in this case. Even body odour is a trigger. I was standing in a shop recently. There were three fat women looking at greetings cards and blocking the way to the counter. As I stood there waiting for them to move, my breathing suddenly became very difficult as the body odour smell was so strong. I had to rush out of the shop and get to my Ventolin as soon as I could.

The list seems to be endless. I have noticed that even the food I eat sometimes provokes an attack. Hot, spicy food is the worst. Any foods containing chilli or a lot of pepper produces an allergic response in me, too, and I have difficulty breathing. Cold air and sea air irritates me too.

I'm on edge all the time trying to avoid trigger factors, and when other people don't show any understanding it makes life even more difficult.

One of the worst triggers of all is cigarette smoke. Even the smell of stale cigarette smoke is irritating. I have banned people from smoking in my house – some people don't like this very much which I find amazing. No one is allowed to smoke in my car. My sister-in-law is understanding and when she wants to smoke during a visit she will sit in the outside loo no matter what the weather. I'm also amazed at people's reactions when I tell them that I've read that only 15 per cent of the smoke produced by a cigarette is inhaled by the person who is smoking it. I know they think I'm ex- aggerating but I'm not. Passive smoking is a real problem for someone who has asthma. I really resent the fact that all that smoke comes my way.

Having to avoid cigarette smoke has restricted my social life even though now there does seem to be more awareness of the problems of smoking and air pollution, and places do now have no smoking areas. But in my case that's still not enough because I can't even get a whiff of smoke. I know some people don't understand when I say that I can't meet them in a pub or anywhere where there may be smokers. But my doctor has warned me that it's essential I keep away from a smoky atmosphere.

Cigarette smoke can cause an asthma attack or other allergic reactions such as irritated eyes, runny noses or even sore throats. It is not surprising that this should be so as cigarette smoke causes a mild though chronic (continuous) inflammation of the lining of the nose, throat and lung airways. This makes the now 'rough- ened' surface far more likely to pick up any passing in- fection or any passing allergen. In someone who already has an allergic type of eczema, cigarette smoke is even more likely to provoke asthmatic problems. Cigarettes are thought to be one of the worst pollutants we can come across, containing hydrocarbons, carbon monox- ide, nicotine and nitrogen dioxide, and they are a great problem because socially the smoke can be difficult to avoid, as only about a quarter is inhaled by the smoker.

The British Allergy Foundation points out that ciga- rette smoke has indeed been reported to increase the risks of allergy in some people. But not only asthmatics can be irritated by cigarette smoke. Even some smokers find that if they are in a crowded room or pub, where lots of people are smoking, they too can be affected by itching, streaming eyes.

Lesley, a thirty-four-year-old reporter, now deliber- ately avoids cigarette smoke in public places because of the effect it has on her. Cigarettes also caused her to resign from her job on a women's magazine.

I didn't realise that it was cigarette smoke that produced such severe reactions in me. I have never ever smoked myself and have to admit that I don't like the smell of smoke, nor do I particularly approve of smoking. It just seemed when I was in my teens and early twenties that whenever I went to a nightclub I ended up not being able to stay for very long. My eyes would quite soon begin to feel really dry and scratchy. If I went home at this point I would be OK. Sometimes I didn't because I was having a good time and I can remember quite a few occasions when my eyes then began to stream so badly I could hardly see. This was compounded by all the tears mixing with my mascara and really stinging – which made my eyes stream even more. This then all ran down my face and I would end up looking like a total mess so I had to go home anyway.

This reaction also happened to me in restaurants several times if they were particularly smoky. I used to get so annoyed that I couldn't even go out for a pleasant dinner without someone else's cigarette smoke ruining my night. I find that's not so bad these days because more and more restaurants have non-smoking tables. Although I have been in a couple of restaurants where the non-smoking table we were asked to sit at was on the edge of the non-smoking area and right next to a smoker's table. That really did make me angry and I asked to be moved as soon as I noticed the fact.

Working with smokers became quite a bind for Lesley and she was angry that she had to leave her job and seek employment elsewhere because of the physical effects on her.

I had worked with smokers before without too much bother. I made sure I didn't sit too near them and if they seemed to be having a few more cigarettes than normal on a particular day I could politely point this out and ask if they could 'ease off' a bit. The situation was helped because there was another woman in my department who hated cigarette smoke and she used to make quite a bit of noise about it.

But when I got a job on another magazine the problem became much worse. To cut a long story short, I only worked there for two months and one of the main reasons I left was that there were two chain smokers in the office who didn't seem to care a hoot about how much they were polluting the air for other people. You'd get into the office early in the morning before other people arrived, but one of the smokers used to get in very early too and even at, say, 8.30 in the morning the office would be filled with a kind of smog. It was disgusting. The whole time I worked there I had sore eyes, my nose felt very irritated and by the end of each day I had a sore, dry throat. It was ridiculous. And as well as the allergic reaction my clothes and hair absolutely stank. By the time I got home the symptoms would begin to subside, but I knew the next day they would just start up again. There was no option really but for me to leave.

4: ANIMAL ALLERGIES

My postbag tells me that sensitivity to animals is a fairly frequent problem. I'm sure most people know of someone who is allergic to cats or dogs. But some people are allergic to any sort of hairy animal, although it's not so much the fur that causes the problems but the tiny scales of skin, called dander. Symptoms of animal allergies can include rashes, itching, streaming noses, watering eyes and even difficulties in breathing. Some figures suggest that a third of allergy patients react in some way to furry animals.

Worried parents with an allergy to pets often ask whether this automatically means that their children will be the same. But people usually inherit the tendency to allergy rather than the specific allergy itself, so my response is that it doesn't necessarily mean that pets will be a problem for the children. However, if the parent's reaction is a very strong one, or the children show any sign at all of developing an allergy, then it's always wise to seek your doctor's advice.

I'm also asked whether or not pet birds can cause such an allergic reaction, or whether pets such as hamsters, guinea pigs, rabbits or gerbils can create allergens. The answer is yes. Children who suffer from asthma may have to be careful to avoid such pets at home or even in school.

I have also been asked whether an animal's saliva can trigger allergic symptoms but I've never heard of anyone reacting in this way. Indeed, dogs' and cats' saliva is not too different from our own in composition, so I wouldn't expect it to be a specific allergen.

With pet allergies sufferers often don't even have to come into contact with the allergen for very long, their reactions appearing within minutes. Such sufferers should not, of course, keep any pets.

CATS AND DOGS

Some people have discovered that they are allergic to certain breeds of cats, which is the case for Joy, who also suffers from hay fever.

> Cats make me get very short of breath and make me sneeze. If it's a long-haired pedigree cat the reaction can happen very quickly. I don't seem to react too badly to an ordinary moggy. A friend has a Blue Persian cat and I can't be in the same room for more than half an hour even if I don't touch it. Yet cats seem to know I have an allergy to them, because I could be in a roomful of people and a cat will come in and head straight for my lap! If I do touch a cat and then touch my eyes they itch for ages.

Spending a lot of time with cats and dogs as a child does not make you more likely to develop this allergy. If someone is susceptible to allergies, then early exposure could increase the likelihood, but if you're not susceptible then it won't cause any problems.

As with most allergies, the degrees to which people are affected can vary. While some people can quite happily visit friends who have pets, provided the animals are taken out of the room, others find that removing the pets makes no difference whatsoever.

Mike, who spoke about his perennial rhinitis on page 18, cannot tolerate any contact with cats or dogs.

> When I lived in Kenya as a child at about the age of nine, we had two dogs. They were a cross between an Alsatian and a Rhodesian ridgeback. When they were puppies they used to live inside the house but they slept in a utility room.
>
> My brother and I were given the responsibility of looking after the dogs since they were given to us as presents. It's only looking back that I can see the pattern of my allergic reactions developing.

I used to start sneezing when I had close contact, such as playing with them or going into their room. We had to clean up their mess every morning when they were puppies. I used to sneeze and then be sniffly on the way to school in the morning. I didn't realise that I had an allergy. I just thought that I had a continuous cold. I didn't know any better and my parents didn't think much more of it than that I was a bit of a sniffly sort of kid.

A few years later we moved to the West Indies. We had another dog here but again because of the climate he stayed outside. He was a beautiful golden Labrador called Sandy.

It was around this time that my parents went as far as taking me to an ear, nose and throat specialist to see what was wrong with me and to find out why my nose was constantly blocked. He had a quick look at my nose and apparently I had a deviated septum. But he said it wasn't bad enough to warrant an operation to correct it and that it wasn't necessarily the cause of my problem nor would it be preventing my sinuses from draining properly. He asked whether we thought I was allergic to anything but we said no, because we still hadn't made the connection with animals.

There was always a neighbour's cat who would visit our garden, an ordinary ginger; sometimes I would pick it up or it would jump on my lap. It was then, for the first time, I noticed a definite reaction. Because of the climate you'd be sitting in just swimming trunks and that was when I had direct contact with the cat. I picked it up on my lap and noticed that I had a red spotty and itchy rash on my belly where the cat had been sitting. I became really sniffly and my nose ran, my eyes also became itchy – with hindsight it was much worse than it had been with dogs.

That was the first time Mike and his parents recognised that he must have an allergy to pets, rather than just being a kid who was always catching colds.

That was when we finally made the connection between animals and my symptoms – and that I was worse with cats rather than dogs. We'd been slow to make the connection because our pets had lived outside in the warm climate. They had their own dog house and didn't used to come inside our homes. Even now if I am outdoors with dogs it doesn't really affect me unless I touch them – whatever it is that irritates seems to get blown away by the wind.

Once I realised I had a violent reaction to cats I had to avoid them. I also avoided touching our dogs and we immediately noticed the difference and how much the sniffling stopped.

As a child this was upsetting for me because I was really fond of Sandy. It was awful not being able to play with him so much.

A couple of times I tried playing with cats and the dog. I didn't want to accept that was the way I was and that I would have to give up contact with pets indefinitely. But sure enough as soon as I started to play with animals I would get the same reaction.

Mike admits that one of the most irritating things about coping with his allergy was having to put up with family visits to cat and dog owners' homes.

For many years I would put up with this and accept it as my bad luck and just sniffle away. Over the years, however, my allergy seems to have become even worse. As a teenager I would just sit trying to put on a brave – red – face, together with enduring a runny nose and itchy eyes.

I'd feel embarrassed and I wouldn't want to say to my parents let's go home I'm miserable. So I'd just put up with it. My allergy also got to the stage where if I was in a home, and I didn't know that they even had pets, my reaction would start and I could tell according to the severity of the reaction what sort of animals there were, whether they had cats or dogs, or both. If it was a dog the reaction would build up slowly over a longer period. In cats, I'd pick it up from a settee or something. I'd start streaming much more quickly and the reaction is much more severe.

But what became more and more irritating for me was that once my parents' friends realised the state I was in and were told of the cause, they would make a fuss and take the pets out of the room. I hated attention being drawn to me in this way and putting the animals out didn't make any difference anyway.

When people knew in advance that I was coming they would also put the animals outside and give the house a good hoover. But no matter how well a house had been cleaned and dusted there would always be particles in cushions, furniture, or even curtains, and I would react just the same.

Although Mike managed to avoid cats and dogs in most instances as he grew older, he has been caught out a few times.

I remember one holiday I went on with friends, to a cottage in Scotland. I couldn't stop sneezing and it was only about two days later that a friend admitted that the owners had cats – although the cats hadn't been there for some weeks. For the rest of the week's holiday I couldn't go into the living room and spent my cosy evenings in the kitchen where my symptoms weren't so bad.

One incident finally proved to be the last straw. I went to a friend's wedding in Wales where I had to stay overnight. The reception was held on her parents' farm in Pembrokeshire. The reception was in a marquee outside so all day I felt fine. It had been arranged that I'd be staying in a spare room in the farmhouse.

I went to bed late at night and just crashed out. After a short while I began to get my usual strong reaction to cats although I was puzzled because I hadn't seen any cats all day. But I thought there wasn't much I could do about it at that stage. I didn't want to wake people to find out where the nearest bed and breakfast was and as I was in the middle of nowhere I couldn't have driven – I was rather under the influence of alcohol as well. Anyway it ended up that I didn't sleep all night and by the morning I could hardly breathe. I went down to breakfast looking like some sort of diseased animal, with puffy eyes, a red nose and wheezing as I tried to speak. It turned out that the parents did have cats – seven of them, three long-haired ones, and they had been put in my room during the wedding reception to keep them out of the way!

That was quite a turning point for me. I decided after that I would not put up with uncomfortable symptoms just for the sake of being sociable or not wanting to spoil the party. Grinning and bearing things only meant that I would become even worse.

I've tried taking antihistamines. They either make me drowsy or I feel as if all my symptoms are just being suppressed and are just building up pressure inside my head. That sensation is almost as bad as the original symptoms.

Avoidance is quite straightforward. I'm getting better at telling people and being straight about the problem. I ask people to my house rather than visiting them in their own house. I've learned with age and with more self-confidence to become less tolerant. I've reached the point where I don't care what other people think.

But even with this conscious decision not to put up with things, I've still been caught out. Recently we went to a surprise family anniversary party. Again it was in the middle of nowhere and the owner of the house I was staying in had two brown Labradors which I didn't realise until I got there. I was assured that they weren't allowed upstairs. (I don't really think, as it turned out, that this was the case.) When I tried to sleep the same thing happened, except this time I got straight out of bed and went to a £60-a-night hotel just to avoid a repeat of the seven-cat incident. I'm sure some family members thought I was overreacting. But what people fail to realise is that when I am bad it can take me a few days to recover and for my nose to stop feeling irritated and swollen.

HORSES

Not only cats and dogs cause problems. Many people can have an allergy to horses – although often they aren't even aware of this because we just don't come into contact with horses as often as our favourite domestic pets.

Elizabeth, a thirty-five-year-old word processor operator, had a violent reaction to horses on a family camping holiday when she was fourteen years old, which was very frightening for her and the rest of the family.

We'd been pony-trekking all afternoon. It wasn't the first time I'd been on a horse. But it was the longest time I'd spent on horseback at one go.

When we got back to the tent my eyes began to swell so much I looked Oriental. They also started to itch like mad. My chest began to feel very tight and it was difficult to breathe. Then at about the same time I began to get very red bumps on my chest and face. They were very hot and made my skin feel uncomfortable.

It had been a very hot dusty day and the horse had been sweating and I'm sure that had something to do with it.

I was getting quite panicky but fortunately my aunt was with us and she was a nurse. She realised it was obviously an allergic reaction and she gave me some antihistamine tablets. I'm pretty sure they were Piriton. The tablets made me really sleepy. I slept for about three hours and when I woke the symptoms had 'mysteriously' vanished.

I knew if I came into close contact with a cat it would provoke a slight allergic response. It was only when I stroked a cat and then touched my eyes without washing my hands that it would make my eyes itch. I had no idea horses could cause such a reaction.

I tried riding again several times since that, during the winter, without suffering any effect. Yet when it comes to the summer I have exactly the same reactions, particularly when it's a hot, dry, dusty kind of day, which is a nuisance because I love riding. But I find it's not worth risking such unpleasant results.

INSECT BITES AND STINGS

Creatures that sting do so to protect themselves; insects that bite do so to feed. With mosquitoes, midges and horseflies it is only the female that bites; she needs the blood that a good bite gives her in order to rear her young – no consolation to us as we scratch away!

But whether the attack takes the form of a bite or a sting, the result is the same: a hot, red, swollen, itchy area and, sometimes, more serious consequences. In the case of a sting, the symptoms are the result of the body's reaction to the poison injected; with a bite, they are due to an anti-clotting substance in the insect's saliva which it injects to make the blood flow more easily as it feeds. Although not poisonous, this substance can provoke an allergic-type response around the bite and occasionally throughout the body. Fortunately, mosquitoes in Britain do not carry disease.

When you are bitten early in the season, you're more likely to react and find yourself scratching than you are later on in the summer. This is because your body gradually develops some tolerance, particularly to your local gnats and midges. However this will not help you when you visit a different area and get bitten by an unfamiliar species!

Some people seem to be more attractive to insects than others and individuals differ in how much they react. Elaine, a fifty-five-year-old nurse, found that whenever she went for a summer evening stroll with her husband, or members of her family, she would be the one to be covered in gnat bites, while the others would escape bite-free. She found whatever tolerance she might have developed was totally wiped out when she went on holiday a few hundred miles from her home.

I remember one summer holiday when I was really bad. We had gone to the north of Scotland and stayed in a caravan in Ullapool. We'd been out all day walking in the hills and wandering around a loch. I'd been totally unaware that I'd even been bitten. I certainly didn't feel anything biting me at the time.

It was only in the evening when I started to itch that I realised what must have happened. Every part of my skin that had been exposed was covered in gnat bites: my face, legs, arms. Even my scalp had been bitten. Once the itching started, the bites also began to swell. They must have swollen to about two inches in diameter. I really looked a sight. As I am a nurse I didn't panic because I realised that it was an allergic reaction to the bites.

I also tried hard not to scratch the bites because the last thing I wanted with all those bites was to have infection set in. All we had in the caravan that night was bicarbonate of soda which I mixed to a paste with cold water and put on the bites to try to ease the itching. Of course, the next morning I headed straight for the chemist and bought some antihistamine cream. Even so I was pretty uncomfortable for about two days. And never went anywhere without insect repellent after that.

Some people are actually allergic to the venom of wasps or bees. It produces such a violent reaction that the consequences can prove fatal (see page 85).

5: FOOD ALLERGIES

The role of food in allergy is cause for much debate but, even so, it is one of the main triggers in some sufferers. 'True' allergic reactions to food are due to naturally occurring products such as milk and other dairy products, eggs, fish, shellfish, wheat and the pea and bean family. Some people discover that they even have an allergy to alcohol and vinegar. Reactions usually include some form of urticaria (see page 73) but many experts believe other symptoms such as lethargy and even depression can result. These phenomena are rarely able to be attributed to a specific allergy.

Julia, a forty-two-year-old complementary health therapist, has endured an allergy to eggs since she was a baby.

> I still react very badly to eggs. I was a few months old and when I think about it now, I believe that I was probably exposed to too much egg at that time. I had whooping cough when I was a few months old and had been very poorly. Apparently it was an old-fashioned idea that if you'd had whooping cough you needed to have your strength built up again by being fed with eggs. So I was constantly given raw egg yolk on a spoon.
>
> But I kept on being poorly and sick. I was losing even more weight and this went on for a couple of months. On this particular day I had just been sick all over my mother, just before the doctor was due to arrive. She had gone upstairs to change and came down wearing a yellow sweater. I'm told that when I saw the colour of the sweater I shuddered. The doctor wondered whether the problem was the egg yolk they'd been giving me. Well, they stopped the egg yolks and I was fine after that.

It is worth pointing out here that although Julia blames her allergy on the extra eggs she was fed as a child, this is not likely to be the real reason. The amount of allergen we are exposed to seems to be less important than the susceptibility to develop such an allergy. It is likely to have been a tendency in her genes that was the real culprit.

Julia feels that when she was a child some relatives thought her mother was over-indulging her by not forcing her to eat eggs, and would 'secretly' give her something that perhaps might have an egg glaze.

When this happened I'd have a violent reaction and would always be very sick. As I child it was very difficult at times. I knew I had to avoid eggs – when they looked like an egg – but I didn't know at that age that egg could be present in so many things like a cake or some mayonnaise in a ham and salad sandwich. I always seemed to end up being really sick after going to a birthday party.

Once egg had got into my system I would be very unwell for about twenty-four hours. I had very bad griping pains, I'd feel washed out and exhausted. It might be forty-eight hours before I felt completely normal again.

There have been times when even the smell of eggs has provoked a reaction. Then I got asthma when I was twelve or thirteen.

On one day I decided it was not going to overtake me completely. I remember standing in the garden looking through the window at my mother boiling an egg and just by doing that I had an asthma attack. After that, because I felt it was partly psychosomatic, I turned it around and thought that if I could think myself into it I could think myself out of it. And that has helped over the years. Keeping calm during an asthma attack definitely helps you deal with it.

Julia finds the severity of her reaction to eggs depends on her physical well-being. When her health isn't at its best she only has to touch a foodstuff containing egg to provoke a reaction.

It really does depend on how well I am in myself. I can rub some sauce containing egg on my hand and I get an itchy

rash. When I cook eggs for my son I wear rubber gloves.
I'm quite worried that there's a strong chance he'll pick up
the allergy from me but so far he shows no sign of it. I have
to be very careful when I prepare eggs for him because if I
touch an egg and then touch my eyes they react by swelling
up. I have had throat swellings and I can't swallow and feel
as if the air passages are closing up. Years ago I was told it
was all in the mind. A lot of it is, in a way, in that if you can
keep calm you can deal with it a lot better.

While egg is her main food allergy Julia has since found
out that avocados can produce similar allergic reactions.

I found out about avocados relatively late. I didn't eat them
until I was an adult. I started to eat them and felt that there
was something I didn't quite like about them. When I
began to eat them more often they made me come out in
red weals. So now I avoid avocados too. If I eat a tiny piece
I don't think it would have too disastrous consequences,
unlike eating an egg.

I'm also sure if I ate enough peanuts I would have an
allergic reaction. I don't like the taste of peanut butter very
much and when I have eaten it, which is rarely, it has made
my throat feel itchy.

Food allergies have made Julia very careful because
she's even had to rush to hospital on some occasions
when she has unknowingly come into contact with egg.

I've had to go to hospital a couple of times and been given
adrenaline to counteract the reaction. I do have to be so
careful. Yet it can be very upsetting when you go to a
restaurant and you specifically say that you're allergic to
eggs and ask whether things contain egg and they don't
really take you seriously. I was once in a restaurant and
there must have been coleslaw at the side of the plate.
Rather than preparing me a fresh salad they must have just
taken it off before serving it. I was really ill after that.
Another time a neighbour cooked a meal and part of the
meal was made in a frying pan in which she had previously
fried an egg and I even reacted to that.

I make myself sick if I've unwittingly eaten anything containing egg. I find that works better for me. I can't be doing with twenty-four hours of feeling awful any more. These days people are more aware of allergies and I do think they take you more seriously. But it's still difficult to relax and enjoy your meals when you have to do things like that.

Prawns and strawberries are very common triggers of allergy and reactions such as urticaria. Recently I had a letter from a young man who wondered whether he was allergic to prawns because the first time he'd ever eaten them he had been violently sick. Friends told him that it was probably simply because he'd eaten a 'dodgy' one. But the second time he had prawns the same thing happened again; in fact, he was so ill, he can't even think about prawns without feeling sick.

I had diarrhoea and vomiting for three days. I couldn't stop being sick. It seemed as if all my insides were coming out. I couldn't even keep a glass of water down. I was like this for three days and I felt so dehydrated at the end of it. And by the third day I also felt as if I had nothing left inside me. I felt dreadful – I just sat on the loo and didn't know which end was going to empty first. I had a pink rash on my arms and legs. I had a fever as well just to make matters worse. Could it be that I have an allergy to prawns or was it just bad luck?

It sounds to me that his friends were right – he'd eaten a dodgy prawn and therefore swallowed a large dose of food-poisoning germs with their toxin. But we'll never know for sure, since it's almost certainly too late now for investigations to be successful. Since prawns are by no means essential for our diet, it's probably better for this young man to be safe and just avoid them in the future.

Elaine, who spoke about her allergic reaction when she was covered in gnat bites (see page 38), also finds that summer poses another problem – strawberries.

Initially I didn't realise that strawberries had an effect on me. I do suffer from vertigo occasionally but a couple of years ago I noticed that I seemed to get it more in summer months than during the rest of the year.

A friend called to see me one day just after I was getting over an attack of vertigo. She immediately asked me whether I had been eating strawberries because her husband found that if he ate them, he would inevitably get vertigo. That was when I realised that there was a link. I had been eating strawberries. I now try to avoid them even though I really enjoy them. I know if I did eat any as soon as I opened my eyes the following morning everything would whirl. When I get vertigo it's really difficult to get out of bed. If I do, I lose my balance and I can't see properly. I have to close my eyes and feel my way to the bathroom before getting back to bed and staying there with the help of some medicine for vertigo such as Stemetil.

Citrus fruits seem to create problems for some people, too. I once spoke to someone who couldn't understand why every Christmas she would develop an irritating rash behind her ears and on her face. The rash would consist of hundreds of minute blistery-type spots which would also make her skin feel very hot. After talking to her for a few minutes and asking what foods she regularly ate in abundance at this time of year, it transpired she was very fond of satsumas, clementines and tangerines. It is claimed that it is the juice that causes such reactions – orange in particular – although no one knows what the precise trigger in the juice is. Orange may be the most common culprit simply because we drink more of it than other citrus juices.

Another common allergen is the nut. Peanuts in particular are causing concern at the moment. They, like shellfish or fish, contain proteins which seem particularly liable to become allergenic. No one knows precisely why.

Some experts believe that as a nation we are eating more peanuts than ever before, and are therefore more likely to hear about allergic reactions. It's now thought that something like one in a hundred food allergics are sensitive to peanuts. These nuts can produce violent reactions and even cause death in some cases, although no one knows why. And in some instances you do not even have to swallow a nut to provoke fatal consequences.

Indeed, it is possible to get quite violent reactions even when nuts have only been used in the cooking. Specialists who have observed such potentially tragic reactions want peanuts removed from those dishes where they are not essential to the flavour. Such dishes include curries, chilli dishes and some cakes. Where peanuts are needed, then it should be clearly pointed out both in the name of the dish and in a warning. As peanut reactions are more severe than the worst of the bee and wasp stings – and more likely to end in tragedy – I have to agree with them. Also anyone with an allergy to peanuts should certainly avoid *all* nuts just to be on the safe side.

FOOD INTOLERANCE

Generally, people tend to be rather confused about the difference between an allergy and an intolerance, sometimes also called a 'sensitivity'. For a definite *allergy* to be diagnosed, the presence of a 'hostile' chemical in the body – an antibody – has to be confirmed. An intolerance is not associated with a definite measurable chemical reaction, but the effect it can have via the automatic (autonomic) system can be much the same, though there are not always the common allergy symptoms such as rashes or breathing difficulties or anaphylaxis. An intolerance to a certain food will normally lead to vomiting only minutes afterwards. Peristalsis (the movement of food through the digestive system) will also quicken, leading to diarrhoea.

I once received a letter which told me that if the writer's daughter drank cow's milk rather than soya milk she became violently ill. The writer wanted to know whether this condition affected adults too? The intolerance isn't uncommon among children but, fortunately, it's much rarer in adults – often because they've learned to avoid milk throughout their lives, although it can develop in later life as our case study on page 48 shows.

The condition is likely to be due to a reaction to the proteins in milk or to the fats – called fatty acids – or even to the milk's sugar (lactose). Symptoms can include vomiting, diarrhoea, and sometimes asthma, skin hives or eczema. Some doctors also link it with a failure to grow properly, though others are sceptical about this. Fortunately, it's usually only temporary and should settle if substitutes – such as soya milk – are given instead. Wyeth Nutrition, among others, make an infant formula from vegetable fat soy protein for children with cow's milk allergy or lactose intolerance, which is available from pharmacies.

Lactose intolerance is a fairly common problem, causing cramping pains, wind and a bloated stomach. Sometimes it can make people feel sick with no apparent cause. If these symptoms fall into a pattern and you find that they occur after you have had some milk, then the problem could be lactose intolerance, which means you are unable to digest milk. The condition is thought to affect up to one in ten people in the UK. Yet lactose is contained in many foods apart from the obvious, such as cow's milk, goat's milk, breast milk, cream, yoghurt and vanilla ice-cream. You'll also find it in instant potato, most breads and pastries, powdered eggs and many instant foods and meals, which emphasises yet again the importance of proper food labelling. Some tablets, capsules and medications also contain lactose as a binder or filler.

Maggie, thirty-seven, a student teacher, has suffered from lactose intolerance for the past five years.

It's different to an allergy because I don't burst out in spots or in an itchy rash or anything. The lactose just hurtles straight through me and my body gets rid of it as fast as it can because my body just can't tolerate it.

I first developed the intolerance about five years ago

about six months after my twin daughters were born. I had symptoms of a bloated stomach and severe diarrhoea for no particular reason. I'd be going to the loo about five or six times a day. The intolerance seemed to creep up on me but because I was so busy looking after the twins I didn't notice that something was really wrong.

I was referred to a consultant who tested me for lactose intolerance in order to rule it out – and the test came back positive.

For the first six weeks after diagnosis Maggie was put on a diet containing no milk products at all.

It was just before Christmas; it was horrendous. I couldn't find much to eat at all. There is whey or lactose in some form in all sorts of things, in baked beans, canned soups. The only spread I could find was a Jewish kosher one. I had to drink black tea and coffee. I was really worried because at that time I couldn't find a calcium tablet that wasn't derived from calcium lactate. It's not good for a woman of my age suddenly to stop having calcium in her diet because of the risk of osteoporosis. I've since found one called Calcia which is made from calcium carbonate. I tried soya milk but couldn't tolerate that either.

Maggie's twins also developed lactose intolerance when they were about eighteen months old, which lasted for about two years.

I took them off milk but I left them on small amounts of cheese and was told this was the right thing to do so that they could keep the slight tolerance they had going. And they're fine now.

If you think about it, our bodies aren't really designed for drinking milk the way we do. We're the only animals who keep drinking milk which is designed as a food for the young. Some Asians who don't drink milk often find they are lactose intolerant.

Another condition which sometimes causes confusion is Coeliac disease. Sharon, a twenty-four-year-old PR manager, has severe headaches, chronic diarrhoea and a swollen abdomen if she eats anything containing wheat. Again this is not an allergy to wheat but an intolerance of gluten which is a protein found in wheat, barley, rye and oats.

> I am very careful about avoiding all sorts of foods that contain gluten. I can't eat anything which contains flour, like bread and cakes. My main problem is going to a conference with work and finding a buffet table of food. I have to be very careful about the foods I can take from it.
>
> I have to be so careful – for example, certain brands of baked beans include gluten and some don't. Sometimes manufacturers can change their ingredients. I can take rice and plain vegetables and I can make my own sauces. You can also buy gluten-free products from chemists and some you can get on prescription. If I do eat something containing gluten the unpleasant symptoms can last from a week to eight weeks.

An extreme example of food intolerance to a natural product is a disease known as phenylketonuria, in which the body cannot deal with the amino acid, phenylalanine. Today all children are routinely screened at birth for this problem. If detected they are put on special diets which exclude phenylalanine.

It's important to realise that if you think you may have a food intolerance, medical help should be sought. You should never try to diagnose it yourself. You need to have medical advice from your doctor as well as from a dietician to be sure of an accurate diagnosis and proper treatment.

ADDITIVES

For some years now additives in our food have been blamed for, among other things, urticaria, asthma, general weakness, blurred vision, depression and hyperactivity in children.

'Why do we need food additives?' I am asked. In

brief, the several thousand additives in use (which are often referred to by their 'E' numbers) have been introduced into our diets for a variety of reasons. For example, the acids, such as ascorbic acid, which can be added to fruit juice to delay discolouration, or the acidity regulators such as trisodium citrate, or the antioxidants, BHA or octyl gallate, added to fats to stop them going sour or stale when exposed to air.

Food colourings have been added to many types of food from coloured fizzy drinks to fruit squashes, sweets, jellies, sausages, biscuits, even chewing gum, to make their colour more appealing. Colours used include caramel, riboflavin, annatto and turmeric. In some countries certain food colourings are banned, particularly a yellow food dye called tartrazine. Tartrazine and a dye called sunset yellow have been blamed for allergic reactions such as skin rashes and even asthma.

Preservatives are found in many foods – and sometimes they are vital for keeping the food safe by delaying deterioration or keeping bacteria under control, e.g. sulphur dioxide or potassium sorbate. Food flavourings can include natural flavourings or a flavour enhancer such as sodium 5-ribonucleotide, or monosodium glutamate which can cause problems for some susceptible people, particularly those who suffer from migraine.

Emulsifiers and stabilisers are found in many foods. Emulsifiers allow oil and water to be mixed together without breaking down separately. Stabilisers are added to slow down the process even further as emulsifiers are unlikely to prevent the 'unmixing' indefinitely. Examples of stabilisers are guar gum, xantham gum which can be found in mayonnaise, for instance, or sodium polyphosphates found in soups.

A browse around supermarket shelves soon reveals how some manufacturers have responded to public pressure and concern about the number of additives in our foods. Many foods are now labelled 'artificial additive-free', 'preservative-free' and so on. So the choice is yours and you can now have more control over the additives that you or your family consume. Although, having said that, it can be a confusing business when some labels say only what that particular manufacturer has added. A can of baked beans and sausages, for example, may list sausages but we don't know what those sausages may have added to them. Or if you've bought an unwrapped loaf of bread in a baker's you're unlikely to know all its ingredients.

Parents often asked me my views on food additives and hyperactive children. The only additive that I am convinced about is tartrazine. Hyperactivity in children is definitely a cause for concern and some professionals believe that several foods and additives can induce the problem. But there seems to be no clear medical evidence to prove this theory. Disturbed behaviour and violent mood swings can be the consequence of a variety of factors.

Some experts believe that, contrary to popular belief, additives only provoke allergic reactions in a minority of people. In general, this is my opinion too. But if you are concerned about additives in your food and you believe they can induce a reaction, then perhaps the best advice is to steer away from processed or ready-prepared products.

CLINICAL ECOLOGY

Some practitioners in the field of allergy, not usually recognised by the National Health Service and therefore practising for private fees, have their own definitions of what constitutes an allergy and what symptoms it can bring on. They claim that many chronic conditions, with apparently unrelated symptoms, are due to allergies and are consequently critical of the traditional therapists within the NHS for not recognising such theories. The conditions they would suggest include catarrh, depression, giddiness, fatigue, flu-like illness, high blood pressure, hyperactivity, migraine, painful joints, muscular weakness including Myalgic Ence-phalomyalgia (ME) and even fits.

As a result, a different specialist area has evolved, often known as clinical ecology. Basically, this involves a series of intensive studies on people's adverse reactions to what are generally seen as common-or-garden foodstuffs.

What is undoubtedly true is that a small number of people do suffer from very distressing symptoms for which no medical cause can be found. And, for some of those sufferers, a practitioner who is well versed in the practice of 'elimination' diets can apparently establish a relationship between certain foods and the symptoms. A diet is then suggested to the sufferer, which avoids all the foods to which they have been found to be sensitive. With luck, there won't be too many of these foods, and the diet will enable the sufferer to remain symptom-free while eating a varied diet which includes all the essential nutrients to stay healthy.

I think it's fair to say that the practice of clinical ecology, as I've described it, is more of an art than a science, but as long as it makes the sufferer feel better and eliminates most of the symptoms, then that's fine. As I've explained, clinical ecology is not a speciality recognised within the NHS, although many family doctors and some hospital consultants will use exclusion diets as part of their treatment within the state health service.

6: ECZEMA AND DERMATITIS

Allergy is thought to play a role in eczema and dermatitis. If you're slightly confused by these terms, it helps to remember that they aren't specific skin problems. Eczema and dermatitis are used as virtually interchangeable terms and generally mean inflammation of the skin. The word dermatitis is the more general of the two descriptions, as it can be used for any inflammation of the skin (the name is derived from Old English – *derma* meaning skin, *itis* meaning inflammation).

Eczema is used as a description of a skin reaction characterised, when seen under the microscope, by water-logging of the top layer of skin – the epidermis. The term is derived from the Greek word eczein, which means to boil or bubble over, so 'eczema' is really quite descriptive. The main symptoms are itching, redness and swelling, accompanied by small blisters which often weep and form a crust. It's thought that as many as one in ten or even two out of ten people suffer from this condition and it can range quite drastically in severity from mild to extreme.

ATOPIC ECZEMA

Atopic eczema is thought to be the result of outside factors combining with a person's inherited tendency towards sensitive skin. It's unusual for this type of eczema to develop in adult life and most symptoms begin to appear within the first two years of a child's life – sometimes as early as six weeks. Initially this type of eczema usually manifests itself on the face, scalp and nappy area, and as a child grows it can develop on the neck, hands, feet, arms and legs. About one child in ten suffers from this condition. Fortunately for many young atopic sufferers, the symptoms clear up as they reach adult life. Other figures suggest that 90 per cent of children with eczema grow out of it by the age of eight.

The symptoms can be caused by an allergy, but before I raise too many hopes, allergy is rarely thought to be the *entire* cause. Allergens that may contribute to an eczema attack include certain foods, house-dust mites, pollen and pets.

In the mid-eighties there was concern about adults, and in particular children, cutting out dairy products because of the lack of hard evidence available on dietary treatment for eczema. Such was the concern that the National Eczema Society commissioned research into this controversial subject. Sixty-eight children and their families helped with the study and the results showed that restricted diets helped only a very few children. So it's certainly not wise to think that by cutting out dairy products eczema will miraculously disappear. Even if it does help ease symptoms, you still need to use emollients (moisturisers), which are essential if your skin is to be kept moist and supple.

If you do intend to restrict the intake of dairy products for yourself or your child *be careful*. Any restrictive regime, particularly when it concerns babies and young children, should be approved by your doctor.

Cutting out dairy products is part of twenty-seven-year-old Tola's approach to the management of her eczema. She believes that coping with the condition is a matter of skin care maintenance and working out what combination of treatments and measures helps you. She's had atopic eczema for the past nine years and says she never goes anywhere without Piriton antihistamine tablets and a tube of emollient cream in her bag.

Antihistamines don't really stop the itching but they make you drowsy and that helps you get some sleep.

I have to be so careful with my skin. It's quite dry anyway. I have to use moisturiser at least twice a day, sometimes more. I once spent three weeks in hospital. There I was given a mixture of liquid paraffin and white soft paraffin because my skin was so dry and it needed something very greasy. I've also used steroid ointments.

But I have found that treatments never cure the condition. They just make it more bearable. I believe dealing with eczema is a question of maintenance. I make sure I always moisturise my skin. Even at work I have to go the loo to undress completely and moisturise my skin once every day. Sometimes I have to do it twice depending on how bad my eczema is.

I've tried a variety of things to help control my eczema as the combination of emollients and steroid creams didn't seem to be improving things. Evening Primrose Oil made a tremendous difference at first. The itching stopped and my skin became smoother. Cutting out dairy products has helped a little. The effects weren't dramatic but enough to make me continue avoiding these products. My skin became slightly smoother. Now I don't eat butter, yoghurt, milk chocolate, cheese, anything with cream or milk or butter in such as cakes. There are so many things which include dairy products in their ingredients.

I think eczema is a multifactoral thing. You have to combine the treatments that seem to work for you.

CONTACT DERMATITIS

Another form of skin allergy is known as contact dermatitis. This has similar symptoms to eczema but is specifically caused by contact with substances to which your skin is sensitive. It's a very common problem. I'm sure many people will have come across some product or substance which has irritated their skin, be it washing powder or other household detergents, or costume jewellery, for example. Something like one in ten British women is allergic to nickel, which is used in frames for glasses, jewellery and metal clothing accessories. Lanolin is another potential irritant, often used in cosmetics and facial cleansing products. These days, labels on many such products specify whether or not they contain lanolin. If your skin is sensitive to it, look for products that are lanolin-free and also avoid any containing wool alcohol.

Mary, a thirty-four-year-old suede and leather designer, recently found that she had to examine all manner of things her young baby came into contact with after discovering the child had an allergy to lanolin. This allergy lasted for just six months, which is fortunate as Mary constantly works with materials that contain the very thing to which the child was allergic.

I make all these lambskin hats and boots for babies and I had used them for my elder child with no problems at all. I never even gave it a thought. So naturally I did the same for the new baby and I would put her in a little lambskin hat. Yet she always had unexplained rashes on her cheeks. With the red rash that would appear around her head, I assumed it was all part of the cradle cap she had. The protector straps of her car seat were also made out of lambskin.

So I was really surprised to discover that my daughter had a very bad lanolin allergy. She had cradle cap, as I've said, which I know is perfectly usual for a young baby. I'd been asking friends what they had used to ease the condition when someone suggested I try E45 cream, which is lovely stuff. It's light and absorbs really well so I thought I would try it.

But the reaction she had to the E45 cream – which I now know contains lanolin – was horrible. We were staying at my mother's house at the time. We called the doctor out at three o'clock in the morning because I was so frightened. Her head was sweating so much I had to keep using tissues to try to mop up the beads of sweat forming on her skull. At the base of her skull two glands came up that looked like peas under her skin. I had no idea what was wrong. It was so alarming.

A locum came out and was very bad-tempered to be bothered for a skin infection. But I was so worried. Her pores had opened up and some germs had got in. That's how she caught a nasty skin infection and had to have antibiotics. When I took my daughter to my regular GP I was told that she had an allergy to lanolin and that she might grow out of it. Once I stopped using lanolin-containing products and kept her away from lambskins her rashes cleared up really quickly.

Since then I've found it amazing how many people are allergic to wool and just how many things contain lanolin. Sudocrem has lanolin in it and I used to use that all the time. During the summer I was surprised to discover that many sunscreens contain lanolin as well. The Body Shop was helpful as they had a list of products that contain lanolin so you can avoid them. I think that manufacturers are wising up to the fact that lanolin is becoming less popular.

And of course, lambskins contain it as there's quite a lot of wool oil left in the skins.

If someone picked my daughter up while they wearing woolly jumpers she'd have a rash on her cheek. My husband and I made sure that we always wore cotton sweat shirts. I was also very careful and made sure she wore no woolly jumpers or didn't come into contact with any. She does seem to have sensitive skin and I still have to be careful about the clothes she wears.

A baby's sensitivity is likely to be due to the fineness of their skin (as its top layer has yet to coarsen), so they are 'closer' to any potential allergen. Also, for the first three months of life its mother's antibodies protect it but then its own immune system slowly develops and takes over.

Cosmetics can prove troublesome for children as well as adults, as Katherine, a thirty-seven-year-old fashion designer discovered when her daughter took part in a nursery nativity play and ended up with red, angry-looking skin on her face.

My two-year-old daughter had her face painted with children's face-paints for the play. She was taking part as a sheep and so had a white face with a black nose. I think the problem probably stemmed from the fact that I left the face-paints on for too long. She must have had them on her face for a total of three hours by the time they were ready for the play, did the play and then came home. I didn't wash it off immediately because I thought I would put her in the bath and wash everything altogether.

It was also quite difficult to remove and I had to rub really hard with soap and water. Initially my daughter's face looked red and blotchy but as the evening wore on her face began to look more and more red. She looked as if she had a bad case of sunburn, although she didn't complain about it and it was obviously not distressing her. Luckily, I had some mild hydrocortisone cream at home and I smoothed that on her face. By the next morning the skin on her face had returned to normal.

Something seemingly as innocuous as a sticking-plaster can provoke an allergic response in some people. Stuart, now a thirty-one-year-old sales consultant, was allergic to plasters during his childhood and until his early twenties, although it's an allergy he has since outgrown.

I can remember the first time a plaster irritated my skin. I was always getting cuts and grazes as a child, like any other I suppose. This particular time I had a cut on my arm and I woke up in the morning with a real irritation. My skin was itching so much I scratched and scratched and eventually opened up the wound again – which defeated the whole point of the plaster. It also made it even more painful than it already was.

In the area where the plaster had been my skin was really red and it was also covered in little bumps which looked like goose-pimples. This happened a couple of times and my skin would calm down again once the plaster was taken off and it was exposed to air. After that I always had to have cotton wool and bandages whenever I cut myself.

By the time I was about twenty I'd rather forgotten about my allergy. I'd cut myself with a knife on my hand when I was chopping vegetables. It was quite a deep cut – I still have the scar – and it wouldn't stop bleeding so I put a plaster on it. Despite all the years that had passed I still had exactly the same reaction, the same goose-pimply rash and the red irritated skin.

I know I've outgrown my allergy because I've since used them a few times without any side-effect. I had a couple of patches of eczema on my fingers and on my ankle. The eczema on my finger had become irritated and was weepy so I put on a plaster to protect it and this time I had no reaction at all.

An allergy to sticking-plaster is common. Indeed, more often than not doctors and nurses will ask you if you react to plaster before they put one on.

Believe it or not, many people are allergic to condoms. This does provoke doubt initially and I remember a letter from one woman who said that she wanted to come off the pill. Her boyfriend wasn't in agreement and the reason he gave was that he wouldn't be able to use a condom or she a cap because he was allergic to the rubber in them. Is this a likely story? she asked me.

In all probability the poor chap *was* telling the truth. A small proportion of those who use a condom or a cap as their method of contraception find that they or their partner suffer from a reaction to one or more of the chemicals that are used in its manufacture – not the rubber itself. The reaction takes the form of a red rash that may cause itching, and can look very alarming.

Fortunately, a doctor will soon recognise the signs of this reaction and, if another form of contraception isn't suitable, may advise the use of a hypo-allergenic condom. These condoms, called Allergy, are made by Durex and are available from your chemist.

It's also amazing just how many people get dermatitis as a result of becoming sensitive to nickel. It can sometimes be difficult to arrive at a diagnosis as the sufferer may have the rash on parts of their body not in direct contact with the nickel. While a rash arising under the trigger article – a ring or a bracelet, for example – may immediately pinpoint the cause, a response elsewhere on the body arises from a different immune mechanism. It will often, as a result, require the opinion of a skin specialist so that a firm diagnosis can be made.

When an industrial irritant is responsible, the diagnosis will usually be fairly straightforward. Doctors who specialise in occupational health will be on the lookout for it, having made a study of such trigger substances, and will be very careful to ensure that industrial processes using such substances provide sufficient protection. This can be achieved by the use of suitable extractor fans and protective clothing, and by the enclosure of the particular process so that it's no longer able to contaminate the working environment.

As I've said, many products that are in everyday use in homes or at work can provoke allergic reactions in those susceptible. For thirty-one-year-old Mark, allergic reactions are proving to be a bit of a mystery. Slowly but surely he is working out what he needs to avoid.

I have allergic reactions to cats, washing powder, shampoo, soap, wool, and certain foods, although I haven't worked out exactly whether it is caused by an additive.

My main problem is catarrh which then blocks my sinuses and gives me headaches and also nausea. Shampoos and soaps will bring me out in a rash. Shampoos affect the back of my neck and soaps I use on my face make it go red and blotchy. I can only use non-perfumed ones. Even then I have to alternate each product. I have to use pure soap which is unscented and additive-free, I can't even use vegetable soaps. I find that I can use coal tar and my skin will be OK, but if I use two bars of that in a row I get a reaction.

Sometimes I can eat things and I get a rash on my body, usually my chest, a rash of red dots, as well as catarrh and nausea. I have to be very careful with dairy products. I find they give me catarrh but they don't give me a rash. I think I might be allergic to mushrooms although I still haven't worked it out exactly, which is annoying because sometimes I can eat them and at other times I can't. That's what makes me think it could be a food additive. I've been given anti-nausea and antihistamine tablets. They do deaden the symptoms but if you take them you are just coping with the symptoms rather than sorting out the underlying cause.

Washing powders bother me too. I can't use a biological one. I have to have a non-biological one. It used to cause flaky, scaly skin on my toes which was very peculiar because it didn't affect the skin elsewhere on my body. My mother took me to the doctor and he told her it was an allergy to biological washing powder. So she stopped using it and changed brands and the problem went away.

Wool tends to give me short breaths and a mild asthma attack. About three or four years ago I noticed that when I was bundled up in the cold weather and walking to the tube station I'd get a feeling of tightness in my chest. I realised that it happened when I was wearing a woollen scarf wrapped around my neck and up to my face. I stopped wearing it and the symptoms stopped. When I wore it again the symptoms returned. In the past, woollen jumpers had made the back of my neck very itchy but I'd thought nothing more about it. By deduction I worked out what was triggering this particular reaction so now I avoid buying woollen jumpers and scarves and try to wear cotton all the time. That's annoying in itself without the hassle of trying to find decent cotton jumpers to wear all year round.

Mark echoes the sentiments of many sufferers who have written to me about allergies. They feel that either people dismiss their problems as being all in the mind or they fail to appreciate how uncomfortable an allergy can be.

When you try to explain to people what sort of reactions you get with different things, they have a vision of someone with hay fever whose symptoms will go for the rest of the year. They don't realise that an allergy can make you feel quite ill all year round. They tend to minimise it. Unless you have had an allergy you don't understand how uncomfortable it can be.

But I even have to be careful about what shampoos I use. I have to swap them around. Sometimes I seem to build up an allergy to something. If I don't react to a shampoo at first, the more I use it the more likely I am to get a reaction. It's as if the allergic reaction seems to build up and I don't understand why this happens.

Mark seems to be increasing his sensitivities the more he uses a likely trigger. This is by no means unknown, but he does seem to be suffering more than most and no one can really say why. As we continue to unravel the biochemistry of allergy in the body we will know more answers. But there are so many potential chemical pathways for allergies that, at present, any explanation reads like a detective story, offering clues but leaving the informed reader to draw their own conclusions.

7: SOME OTHER COMMON ALLERGIES

ALLERGY TO DRUGS

Some people develop allergies to medicines. The older penicillins, for example, were particularly likely to cause a reaction, ranging from puffiness and rashes to full-blown anaphylaxis (see page 72).

Bronwen, a twenty-six-year-old business consultant, discovered she was violently allergic to penicillin when she was five years old after being prescribed it for a sore throat. And she's managed to avoid taking it ever since.

> All I can remember about the incident was being ill and the next thing I can remember is taking antibiotics. I remember waking one morning and seeing big red weals all over my body. They were very painful, especially on the soles of my feet where I recall having two very large swellings. It meant that I couldn't even walk.
>
> I remember my mum taking me to the doctor and stripping me down in front of him, saying, 'Just look at this!' I was mortified. We had no idea what it was although he knew straightaway.

Bronwen has since found out that she also has an adverse reaction to another antibiotic, erythromycin.

> I get uncontrollable diarrhoea so I refuse to let anyone give me a prescription for it. I always mention my allergy to doctors. For things like tonsillitis, which I get fairly regularly, I'll usually have tetracycline which seems to work for me.

Some people can develop an allergy to more than one medicine. Frank, a forty-year-old research manager, has allergies to penicillin, aspirin and another chemical, chlorine.

When I was about thirteen I had a cold and I remember my mother giving me aspirin – I'm sure it was something like soluble Disprin. Within twenty-four hours I was vomiting and I had an itchy spotty rash which appeared in small clusters all over me. My mother was so worried that she called the doctor and he said that it was an allergy to aspirin. It wasn't connected to the cold I was suffering from, but to the treatment!

I can remember quite vividly how my chlorine allergy came about. My school didn't have a swimming pool and we didn't have swimming lessons either, so my parents decided to send me to swimming classes. It wasn't long after my aspirin allergy. I went into the swimming pool which was quite heavily imbued with chlorine. The following morning I woke up with a dreadful rash and swellings. The swellings were all over my body in any areas that seemed capable of such a reaction. My lips were swollen, my eyes were puffy and even my armpits were swollen and, the final insult, my private parts were very uncomfortable. I also had a raised pimply rash which was very itchy. My mother called the doctor around yet again and he said it must be an allergy to the chlorine. It must have been several days before I felt better. I didn't mind too much because I was scared stiff of the water anyway and it suited me that I couldn't have any more swimming lessons. In fact, I didn't learn to swim until I was thirty-three in warm, Greek sea water, which was lovely.

My penicillin allergy developed when I was twenty-three. I was off work with flu-like symptoms and my throat was very bad and the doctor decided to give me penicillin. I had a terrible reaction to it. I had to stay off for another week. The rash stayed for a full week. It was uncomfortable for two days then it just looked terrible. It was all over my body. My boss came round to visit me and when he saw me he didn't want to come near me. I knew the penicillin had something to do with it as soon as it happened. It happened within twenty-four hours just the way my aspirin allergy had. Again I was so sick and covered in a rash. So the doctor came back to see me and told me it was a reaction to the penicillin and that I must be allergic to it. I've not taken it since.

I know I have been in chlorine pools since and it has had no effect. I'm sure the old swimming baths used to be particularly bad. I do make sure I avoid penicillin or aspirin because that's quite straightforward as there are easy alternatives to them. It's not quite the same with swimming pools.

While some people clearly do react against particular medication, it has to be said that many more people will have an emotional reaction to the thought of taking drugs – knowing unconsciously that today's medicines can be very strong indeed and can sometimes cause powerful side-effects.

Many letters from my postbag contain the phrase 'I'm not one for taking medicines.' The writer will see food as a 'safer' treatment and will often ask if I can recommend a diet for what ails them. Sometimes they will be on what I know is a life-saving medicine and they are thinking of stopping it! I give them responsible guidance. I point out that most doctors, unlike those in previous ages, do try to keep prescribing to a minimum. (In previous times there were few effective medicines – the rest were bottles of coloured water. As a result, they rarely, if ever, caused anything – effect or side-effect!)

If your doctor has prescribed medication for you, he or she is confident that the advantages will outweigh the disadvantages. So if you have any worries about your medicines, I strongly recommend you discuss them with your GP.

SUN ALLERGY

The vast majority of people who have this condition, medically known as PLE, polymorphic light eruption, are able to control it by avoiding prolonged exposure to the sun, and by applying high-protection sunscreens, since it is triggered by the sun's ultraviolet rays (though some medicines can trigger it). Dermatologists tell us that PLE is most commonly triggered off by the ultraviolet A (UVA) component of sunlight. Sunlight also produces ultraviolet B (UVB) and visible light. Although UVB rays are far stronger than UVA – UVB being the major cause of sunburn, skin ageing and skin cancer – the actual amount of UVA reaching the earth's surface at midday during the summer is 100 times greater than UVB.

The allergy manifests itself in the form of a rash of red, itchy spots which can turn into watery blisters. Areas most likely to be affected are those that are usually covered in the winter months, such as arms and legs.

In extreme cases, PUVA treatment – which strengthens the body's resistance to sunlight – may be the answer. PUVA is a treatment requiring the long-term use of ultraviolet A light in conjunction with Psoralen, a naturally occurring substance found in certain plant seeds. The treatment can be given by mouth or topically, that is, applied directly on to the skin. A likely candidate for treatment would be someone who, despite sunscreens, is unable to go outside without suffering an allergic reaction to the sun's rays.

PUVA treatment does, however, carry a slight risk of future skin cancer, and all potential patients are asked to sign a consent form before beginning their treatment. However, the risk is no greater than spending two weeks in a very hot climate in the full glare of the sun – something many of us do without giving a second thought to the dangers.

For the minority who undergo PUVA, it is most important to approach it with a sensible attitude. Try not to get impatient – the treatment must be allowed to run its full course for it to have its proper impact. Pace yourself, closely observing your body's reactions. And, as with any medical treatment, talk to the consultant so you understand what it entails.

Like any other sudden-onset skin condition triggered by sensitivity to sunlight, there are many aspects of PLE which are currently unknown to us. For example, we don't know its precise origins, nor why it is more common among young women.

PLE is yet another indication that over-exposure to sunlight is not too good for our health.

SPERM ALLERGY

Couples who have had difficulty conceiving often write to me because they are worried about the possibility of a sperm allergy. I recall a letter from one couple who had been trying for a baby for three years with no luck and had consequently begun fertility investigations. As a result they wondered whether having sex five or six times a week could produce an allergic reaction in the woman to the husband's sperm.

They needn't have worried on that score. You can't make yourself allergic to sperm by frequent intercourse. Either you have an allergy or you don't – and if you did have one any fertility investigation would soon reveal it.

Such a thing as sperm allergy does exist, though. Some women have antibodies in their cervical mucus which fight off sperm, treating them as foreign bodies and so preventing conception. The presence of such antibodies is detected in a post-coital test which is carried out early on in any fertility investigation. Again, frequency of intercourse has nothing to do with it. However, it is worth noting that while it is important to have regular intercourse, particularly around the time you think you are ovulating, some doctors advise against overdoing it during the fertile period. They recommend that you have sex no more than once a day, to ensure that your husband's semen (assuming his sperm count is normal) contains a sufficient concentration of sperm in order to maximise your chances of conceiving.

To overcome this allergy (which brings about the production of antibodies to the sperm rather than the symptoms of an allergy) many couples are advised to use a condom for six months. This is because the source of the antibody is mainly the woman's cervical mucus. This allows the reaction to the sperm, in its absence, to diminish – often making a pregnancy possible again once intercourse without a condom recommences.

One of the most effective ways to deal with the problem these days is the test-tube baby technique, fertilising the woman's ovum outside the body.

YEAST ALLERGY

Some people attribute symptoms of bloatedness, tiredness, cramps and depression to candidiasis, the presence of the yeast candida in the intestines and large bowel. I know of no acceptable proof that this is a probability – but it's regularly claimed so to be. It is suggested that eating live yoghurt helps since it is a rich culture of the friendly bacteria, the lactobacillus, which is said to counter the growth of the candida fungus.

OFFICE BUILDING SYNDROME

This covers a multitude of symptoms which have been put forward by office workers usually after they have moved into an new office building which is 'environmentally controlled'. This means that the air is circulated and filtered, the windows are double glazed and sealed and often there is a constant noise as the air passes through its various conduits and vents.

Fluorescent lighting may be the main light source with little natural light penetrating into the centre of the building. It's a bit like being in a stationary space ship.

The complaints are varied but mainly concern the respiratory system. Inflamed sinuses causing headaches, a tight chest, a constant dry sore nose and throat and a continual feeling of a cold in the head are but a few. Migraines, lethargy, depression, and many variations, are all complaints that I have had in my postbag related to this syndrome. And I have discovered that the individual will usually be convinced that some aspect of the physical environment is to blame, and it's rarely possible to disagree. Indeed, when the well-known reasons for many of these symptoms are put forward by specialists in environmental health, the sufferer will be offended at even a suggestion that there are non-physical provocations to their disease. But this is often what their main complaint is – a lack of ease with their surroundings rather than a specific medical condition.

The inability to open a window when it feels stuffy or to turn the air conditioning off when the background hiss is proving annoying, plus the flickering of the fluorescent lights or the almost unconscious feeling of claustrophobia, are all strong triggers to muscular tension and the mild anxiety which follows. These in themselves can provoke most, if not all, of the symptoms which are regularly complained of.

Suffice to say that enough people who work in such modern buildings have complained of similar symptoms for the syndrome to have become a definite entity, whether the cause is physical or socio/psychological. In my opinion it exists but it is often very difficult to establish the precise cause. Is it an allergy to the dust – small particles of which may be able to be circulated around the building in the air conditioning? Is it an 'allergy' to the 'irritants' being given off by the photocopiers or other equipment?

Once again, the word allergy crops up but many would argue that it is the wrong use of the word. It's likely that the diagnoses of such allergies are more due to art than science.

I remember a colleague telling me that he was asked to adjudicate in a matter where compensation was being claimed on similar environmental grounds. The sufferer had become ill, of that there was no doubt, but was insisting one particular aspect of the environment was the cause. Other doctors had been consulted but could find no cause and effect relationship. My colleague concluded that the sufferer was ill and the 'good' employer agreed to accept the request for compensation for the sickness – even though it was never shown to be their fault. The sufferer refused to accept the compensation saying that it was important that the cause of the illness was accepted, even though all that was asked for was now being offered.

Sometimes there can be few if any conclusions in human affairs.

8: ALLERGY-RELATED ILLNESSES

ANAPHYLACTIC SHOCK

I have often been asked what exactly this term means, and whether it is a condition. Well, it most certainly is. The allergic reaction to the offending substance is so dramatic that the tissues swell, making breathing difficult, the blood pressure plummets, the skin may puff up and be covered in urticaria or hives (see page 73) and the sufferer may also vomit and have diarrhoea. If the condition is not treated immediately with injected adrenaline, and possibly also an antihistamine injected into a vein or even steroids intravenously in very severe cases, the outcome can be extreme breathlessness, gross swelling of the body (particularly the wind pipe), heart failure and death.

This type of shock comes from an extreme sensitivity to a known allergen, for example a bee sting. Such a severe and immediate reaction usually means the offending antigen has been injected rather than eaten, and is more inclined to cause hives and weals or red raised itchy patches on the skin instead of the general body effects.

MIGRAINE

The role of allergy in migraine is another area where opinions are divided. Migraine is usually a one-sided headache, sometimes with other symptoms such as loss of appetite, nausea or vomiting. Some sufferers can have migraine when their attacks are preceded by warning symptoms – called the aura – which may include flashing lights before the eyes, shimmering or double vision, slurred speech, numbness and giddiness. These symptoms are probably due to a sudden constriction in some of the blood vessels within the brain.

The headache comes on as these vessels then begin to expand and the blood surges through, leading to the characteristic throbbing headache. Many experts believe that this constriction and dilation is brought about by changing levels of certain chemicals circulating in the body, such as adrenaline – also released during stress – and prostaglandins. Adrenaline tenses the muscles, the heart and its blood vessels to prepare us for 'fight or flight'. Prostaglandins sensitise the nerve endings to make us more alert. In susceptible people they will 'overdo' it and cause the above symptoms. Studies also suggest that there may be a slight difference – perhaps inherited – in the biochemical make-up of migraine sufferers which makes them more susceptible.

It has been well established that migraine can be triggered by certain foods, although some experts believe that this is true of only one in ten sufferers. So it's important to understand that food is not the main cause of migraine, but it will very often trigger attacks in some people.

Food known to trigger migraines includes chocolate, alcohol (particularly red wine), cheese, citrus fruits, nuts, meats, dairy products, coffee and tea, monosodium glutamate, shellfish and fried foods. Of course, other foods can trigger migraine attacks in individuals; some sufferers have even traced their sensitivity down to the humble onion family, pork, or sharp, unripe green apples, while cutting out wheat-containing products has helped others. It is largely a matter of trial and error and what can affect one person may not cause migraine in another. For some sufferers, food may not even play a part in their migraines at all.

As I mentioned earlier, chemicals added to food can

trigger problems too. Some people find that they develop migraine after eating cured meats or a Chinese meal, where monosodium glutamate is frequently used as a flavour enhancer. This additive is found in many ready-made sauces as well as stock cubes so it's worth spending a few moments in the supermarket checking a product's list of ingredients if you feel monosodium glutamate affects you. In cured meats (this category includes hot dogs, bacon, ham and salami) nitrites, chemicals known as vasodilators which widen blood vessels, may have been added to the salt used in the curing process.

Surprisingly perhaps, ice-cream, too, can give some people migraine. This is to do with temperature rather than content, since a cold feeling on the roof of the mouth can produce referred pain and a headache.

While some sufferers find to their disappointment that food has nothing to do with provoking their migraines, others have been more fortunate and have been able to pinpoint quite accurately what foods to omit from their diet.

URTICARIA

I am often asked what exactly urticaria is. More often known as hives or nettle rash, it is a very common skin condition which affects one in five people at some time in their lives. Women are particularly prone, perhaps because of hormonal influences. With 'ordinary' urticaria, weals – intensely itchy raised marks on the surface of the skin – suddenly develop. They are usually short-lived, lasting for a few hours or days, but may last longer. The weals can be any size, appear anywhere on the sufferer's body and may be numerous. They are usually pale in the middle and red around the edges and are due to dilation of the capillaries which makes their walls more permeable, enabling a clear fluid called serum to leak out. If enough serum leaks out, blisters may form.

If deeper tissues are involved, a more severe type of urticaria, known as angio-oedema, may occur. Then the swellings are much larger, commonly affecting the face, eyelids, hands, forearms and throat and sometimes causing serious breathing difficulties. Joints in the arms and legs may also become inflamed and painful. About half of those people who suffer from ordinary urticaria have recurrent attacks of angio-oedema too.

What causes this reaction in the blood vessels? Often it is due to an increased circulation of histamine – a chemical normally present in the body. This increase can be triggered by many factors, including various foods, drugs and inhalants such as pollens, house dust and animal 'dander'. Two foods that are frequently responsible are shellfish and strawberries – so urticaria is a hazard of summer for those susceptible. Other foods that may produce the reaction include eggs, nuts, chocolate, tomatoes, pork, milk and yeast, as well as artificial colourings and preservatives.

Aspirin can also be a cause of urticaria, or it can aggravate it. Penicillin is another possible culprit, as are the non-steroidal anti-inflammatory drugs often given to treat arthritis.

Sometimes contact with certain substances will bring the symptoms on – cosmetics are one example. Insect stings can also cause this type of reaction, which may even be life-threatening if the breathing is affected.

People whose urticaria occurs in response to triggers such as these are often, but not always, allergy-prone individuals – sufferers from hay fever, asthma or eczema for example – and the tendency can run in families. Anxiety may also play a part. Other constituents in the body – called catechol amines – can, by irritating the tissues surrounding them, have the same effect on the blood vessels as histamine and almost anything can act as the trigger in this allergic-type of urticaria. I once had it after eating raw fish in a foreign restaurant, for example, but that may also have been due to the monosodium glutamate used as a taste-enhancer.

It can therefore be exceedingly difficult to track down the cause if the attacks are recurrent. In fact three out of four people are unable to do so, despite persistent detective work.

Some more unusual forms of urticaria have a physical cause. Cold winds or rain, or just immersing the hands or bathing in cold water, can cause weals to appear in susceptible people. If an ice cube on the skin produces a weal, this confirms the diagnosis of 'cold urticaria' – the type induced by cold temperatures.

Some people develop weals when exposed to sunlight – 'solar urticaria' – deep, painful, non-itchy swellings then occur about two hours after exposure anywhere where pressure is applied to the skin. The hands may swell, for instance, after carrying a heavy shopping bag, or the balls of the feet after spending some time on a ladder.

Another strange form of urticaria is called dermographism, loosely 'translated' as skin writing. A mild, stroking pressure – with a fingernail for example – will produce a temporary, raised line with reddened edges. The skin can literally be used as a drawing board.

Urticaria can occur as part of some other underlying condition, such as thyroid disease. So if the cause is not immediately apparent or you have more than one attack your GP may wish to do blood tests and other investigations or refer you to a skin specialist.

9: HOW TO COPE WITH AN ALLERGY

TREATMENT

It may be helpful when you visit your GP to take a photograph of a particular rash, or perhaps an allergic response that might have caused your lips to swell, for example. Your doctor will be all too aware that identifying allergens is very difficult. He or she will almost certainly ask you whether anyone else in your family has a history of allergic reactions because, as I've pointed out earlier, allergy does have a tendency to run in families. But do be sure to seek your doctor's advice before falling for the lure of a clinic's advertisement that suggests there are 'magic', immediate cures for allergies. I get many letters from people who have been 'ripped off', so you can't be too careful.

In some instances, such as hay fever or urticaria, allergies can be treated with antihistamines. But coping with allergies, as well as treatment, may vary from allergy to allergy, and individual to individual. In the following pages I have dealt with each category separately, but it may be worth your while reading through all the advice because some of the self-help measures advised under each section could also apply to your case.

Hay fever

Unfortunately there isn't one routine or treatment, alone or in combination, which will be the answer for every sufferer. With your doctor's advice you will want to try various options available and find what suits you best.

Do remember that there is no cure for hay fever, although nasal sprays available on prescription are very helpful. Your GP may prescribe an antihistamine nasal spray such as Rhinolast (azelastine hydrochloride) for example, which both blocks the action of the pollen as well as enhancing the effects that the local tissues have in overcoming it. It's a new kind of antihistamine which patients find helpful in easing congestion, sneezing and nasal itching, discharge and swelling.

Steroid drops or sprays could be prescribed. They are thought to be one of the most effective measures when managing an allergy such as hay fever, dampening the allergic response and cutting down on any inflammation and swelling. Beconase Hay Fever (beclomethasone dipropionate), for example, is a popular choice, as is Rhinocort (budesonide). To get the most out of this kind of treatment you need to use the spray regularly and start *before* the season begins.

Mast cell stabilisers which help control nasal symptoms by preventing allergic reactions are another option. Rynacrom Nasal Spray (sodium cromoglycate) can be used to prevent the symptoms of both hay fever and perennial rhinitis developing. Since therapy is essentially preventive, it's important that you maintain a regular dosage rather than using the drops to deal with symptoms once they develop. Side-effects of sprays can be irritation of the nasal mucosa and a taste disturbance. (Sodium cromoglycate and antihistamine eye drops are also available.)

Nasal sprays such as Otrivine (xylometazoline) containing decongestants which shrink swollen nasal tissues can provide relief from a blocked nose, but should only be used in the short term since long-term use may actually aggravate the condition.

Antihistamines can be prescribed for hay fever and there are so many different types available that I don't have space to list them all in this book. An antihistamine such as promethazine (Phenergan) is a powerful long-acting antihistamine with additional anti-emetic (prevents vomiting), anticholinergic (dampens the body's secretion production) and sedative/calming effects. Most common side-effects can include drowsiness, dizziness, restlessness, headaches, nightmares, tiredness and disorientation. Piriton (chlorpheniramine maleate) can also cause drowsiness, impaired reactions and dizziness.

Newer antihistamines astemizole (Hismanal), terfenadine (Triludan or Seldane), loratadine (Clarityn) or acrivastine (Semprex), and cetirizine (Zirtek) can be tried, which don't have the sedative side-effects of promethazine. But care should be taken initially, as with all drugs taken for the first time, because there may be rare cases when the patient reacts badly.

Over-the-counter antihistamine tablets, such as Triludan, Seldane or Aller-Eze, are popular forms of treatment. For best relief, start taking antihistamines as soon as the first symptoms occur, although treatment can be begun at any time.

There are many self-help measures you can take to relieve the symptoms of hay fever. Wearing plain glasses or sunglasses can prevent much of the eye irritation by stopping pollen grains entering the eyes. Keep windows and doors closed, especially when lawns are being mowed. And make sure someone else mows the lawn for you or you're just asking for trouble.

Stay away from pets if they have been outside rolling around in the garden or the park. Try to plan your day to avoid being outdoors in the morning and evening when pollen counts are at their highest. Don't go on country walks and avoid parks or gardens on warm and sunny days, or, if this is impossible, wash your hair afterwards. Keep car windows and air vents closed when you're out driving. Don't smoke, because this causes further irritation to those susceptible to allergies. Buy good quality disposable tissues which are softer and kinder on your nose than rougher ones.

Make sure you check the day's pollen count forecasts.

By doing this you can plan outings to the city centre or the country, avoiding places where you know your hay fever symptoms will be aggravated. If you're not sure exactly what type of pollen triggers your -allergy, it's worthwhile making a note of when your symptoms start, which time of year they are at their worst and when they finally trail off. Tree pollen affects people in spring, grass pollen in early summer, and moulds and fungi spores in the autumn.

And a final word of hope. Most hay fever sufferers do grow out of it eventually.

Perennial rhinitis

Many people who suffer from perennial rhinitis just put up with it; they think the symptoms are too trivial to bother their doctor, or they try to treat themselves with medicines bought from the chemist, such as nasal decongestant sprays. Although these can be all right, used sparingly, for the short-term relief of a blocked nose at the end of a common cold, they are quite unsuitable for treating the long-term blocked nose of perennial rhinitis. Over-use of these sprays will soon damage the lining of the nose and actually make the condition worse with so-called 'rebound congestion'. Antihistamines bought over the counter will temporarily dry up a runny nose, but they will have no effect on a blocked nose and can cause drowsiness.

When nasal symptoms are persistent, it is important to consult a doctor, as there are several effective treatments that can be prescribed once the possible non-allergic causes have been excluded. Obviously, identifying the allergen so that the sufferer can avoid it as far as possible is helpful. Alternatively, anti-allergic, anti-inflammatory nasal sprays or drops, such as sodium cromoglycate (Rynacrom, for example) or corticosteroids, if used consistently as directed, are very effective at both preventing and relieving symptoms. Sufferers often have, or have had, other allergic-type conditions, such as eczema or asthma, or these may run in the family. Successful treatment of rhinitis can also keep asthma attacks at bay.

So it is worthwhile consulting your doctor if you seem to have a permanent head cold or 'hay fever' – these always have a limited duration. Perennial rhinitis does not, but modern treatments will relieve it.

Sufferers of perennial rhinitis should avoid house-dust mites (see pages 82–4), pets and moulds, just as asthma sufferers do. Don't overlook house plants either, their damp soil or compost provides an ideal place for moulds to grow. Carpets shouldn't really be used in bathrooms or kitchens, where they are likely to become damp, thus causing mould to develop.

Asthma

Asthma is, as I've said, surprisingly common and can be treated easily and effectively. Medicines are given to help prevent the symptoms occurring or to give relief when you have the symptoms. Remember that in all cases of asthma, whatever the cause, drugs can be used to great effect. They are mostly taken via an inhaler, which shoots the medication into the area where it's most needed – the breathing passages. Some expand the air tubes, making it easier for the sufferer to breathe, and also reducing the chance of an attack.

The medicines used to treat asthma include bron-chodilators (airway openers) and inhaled steroids. The major bronchodilators are salbutamol (Ventolin, for ex-ample) and terbutaline (Bricanyl), best taken by inhaler (or in the form of an aerosol mist by a nebuliser), be-cause this means that small amounts of medicine reach the airways quickly to relax muscle spasm. You may also be prescribed bronchodilators in tablet or syrup form. Most common side-effects of salbutamol and terbutaline include mild muscle tremor (usually the hands), anxiety and restlessness, cramp and palpita-tions.

Theophylline is another kind of bronchodilator prescribed in capsule, tablet or syrup form (Lasma, for example) which relaxes bronchial muscles. Most common side-effects include nausea or vomiting.

Inhaled steroids (Becloforte and Becotide, for instance) are effective as they help dampen down the irritability of the airways. In standard doses there are relatively few side-effects because of the small size of the doses involved and because, when inhaled, the medicine goes straight to the airways. This lowers the risk of the medicine affecting any other part of the body. Sometimes patients develop a mild throat infection, and occasionally others find that their voice becomes husky. It might help to rinse your mouth thoroughly with water after using such a medicine.

Sodium cromoglycate (Intal, for example) is also used to prevent symptoms of asthma, and may halt the release of certain chemicals which cause spasm. It can also cause throat irritation, coughing and brief bronchospasm. Steroid tablets (Prednisolone, for example) may be needed for severe asthma.

People with asthma have airways which have become over-sensitive. This means that they are red and sore or inflamed most of the time. This, in turn, means that because they are already 'irritated' it doesn't take them long to react to allergens such as animals, cigarette smoke, air pollution, or cold air. When they do react like this, these airways become even narrower. So if you suffer from asthma and know what triggers an attack do try to avoid that trigger.

Try to keep your house as free from dust as possible. The National Asthma Campaign points out that around 60 per cent of all schoolchildren with asthma are allergic to house-dust mite droppings. All allergy sufferers who find that the house-dust mite aggravates them can minimise their problem by hoovering floors and furnishings and damp-dusting frequently, covering mattresses with a plastic cover and using pillows and duvets made from artificial fibres rather than feathers. Polished boards or 'lino' are less of a mite trap than carpets. Mites thrive in warmth, so keep the bedroom cool and well aired. Smaller objects, such as children's fluffy toys, can be put into the deep freeze every so often for about six hours – mites cannot survive at that temperature.

It really is important to wash sheets, pillowcases, and duvet covers at very high temperatures. Newer washing powders and liquids have meant that clothes can now be effectively washed at lower temperatures, but in the case of the house-dust mite the water needs to be pretty hot to kill them all off.

If you find house-dust mites could be aggravating your asthma, eczema or rhinitis, then there are many products, such as zip-up mattress and pillow covers, currently available on the market to help control the problem. These use a system of interliners, made from a special fabric, for mattresses, duvets and pillows, or come ready fitted to a range of beds and pillows, and work by preventing contact with house-dust mites during sleep. The fabric has a unique microporous membrane which allows body moisture and heat to pass through it. The products are fairly expensive though: a double mattress pack, including two pillow interliners, could cost you around £190; mattress, pillow and duvet covers together about £300. However trials have shown that 'allergen exclusion' of this nature can reduce allergic symptoms.

Slumberland, the bed manufacturers, also have a range which incorporates the Intervent technology into mattresses and pillows, which should be available from Slumberland retailers.

Studies show that careful avoidance of the house-dust mite can bring about a significant reduction in the symptoms of allergic airways disease. It's also likely to help sufferers who have sore or puffy eyes first thing in the morning that are not due to an infection.

At home you should keep rooms well aired and try to cut down on condensation wherever possible. If there are any areas of walls with mould growing scrub it away as soon as you notice it, since mould can release tiny particles similar to pollen which could be yet another allergen your body has to deal with.

You shouldn't smoke and you should also avoid passive smoking. It's especially important for children with asthma to avoid cigarette smoke and you should be strict about anyone smoking near your children, particularly visitors to your house.

You could also try using domestic ionisers, which are small electrical appliances that stabilise the negative electrical charges of split atoms floating in the air. Proponents claim that these can 'cure' many symptoms, including perennial rhinitis, sore eyes, and even asthma. However, like most doctors, I'm sceptical.

Even though exercise can bring on wheezing, moderate exercise, such as swimming, should be undertaken, especially by children. Using a bronchodilator drug before exercise helps to prevent an attack.

Always keep your drugs close at hand. That advice goes for children as well, who should have medication with them at school at all times.

Many doctors suggest that the regular use of a peak flow meter can help a sufferer or their carer measure the progress of the asthma. These are simple gauges which, when you blow as hard as you can into them, measure the peak expiratory flow, which is a very good indicator of how well the lungs are functioning. These meters can be prescribed on the NHS.

Don't forget that when you go on holiday you will need to take sufficient supplies with you to cover all eventualities. If you're thinking of going away you should speak to your doctor or pharmacist for advice. You may need to ask him whether your particular medication and the way you use it will need to be handled differently in a hot country, for example. Some means of delivery, such as those used for Rotacaps and Spincaps, may be subject to changes.

Most sufferers or their carers will already know that asthma can be made worse by sudden changes in temperature – either from hot to cold or vice versa. Keep an extra careful eye on young children with asthma if this is likely. Ask your doctor in advance what, if any, increase in dosage of your usual medicines would be wise. Also remember that abroad very different foods may be eaten and, if the sufferer is particularly prone to attack due to dietary changes, try to take a fall-back supply of known, safe foods.

If you feel your asthma is suddenly getting worse you should contact your doctor.

Insect bites and stings

It is wise to use insect repellent if you know you are susceptible to insect bites. In general, insect repellents should protect you for about two hours and, if you are bitten, iced water or witch-hazel, calamine lotion or soothing antiseptic creams available from the chemist will usually calm the irritation. Other over-the-counter remedies tend to be antihistamine medicines, made specifically for bites and stings, to combat any allergic reactions. They can also reduce more severe swelling and irritation and some contain local anaesthetics to ease pain or irritation.

For insect bite reactions your doctor or pharmacist may prescribe creams or ointments containing the mild topical corticosteroid hydrocortisone (Mildison Lipocream, Efcortelan, for example) or a local anaesthetic such as lignocaine (Xylocaine).

However, a few people develop an allergy to wasp or bee stings and can then have an extreme, even life-threatening, reaction which may come on only seconds after the sting. The sufferer may feel dizzy and sick, have runny, itchy nose and eyes and develop a rash.

Their limbs may swell, they may have difficulty breathing and even lose consciousness. If any of these symptoms occur after being stung, it is essential to get to a hospital with an accident and emergency unit (casualty department) or to a doctor *immediately*.

Similarly, for stings in the mouth, multiple stings or if a child under the age of two is stung, it is best to seek medical advice without delay.

For a bee sting, remove the sting with a fingernail by scraping it out sideways and in the direction the sting is pointing, rather than pinching and pulling it out, as this can squeeze the remaining venom into the skin. To counteract the acid in a bee sting, apply ice-cold water containing a little bicarbonate of soda. Wasp stings are alkaline, so bathe them with a little vinegar in ice-cold water. A wasp doesn't leave its sting behind, just a chemical irritant.

Take care when you're out and about. Don't use perfume, hair sprays or aftershave when bees or wasps are around, as they can be attracted by the scent. Bright colours may also attract insects, so wear pale clothes that cover your arms and legs against gnats and midges, especially if you are prone to insect bites.

Examine food and sweet drinks before putting them in your mouth and wipe food from your lips if eating out of doors. I've been badly stung on the top lip by a wasp that, on a hot, dark night, was unseen in a glass of lemonade.

Don't panic if bees or wasps buzz around you and don't hit out at them. Either ignore them or walk away.

Food allergies

Some doctors may want to prescribe capsules of sodium cromoglycate for certain sufferers of food allergy. This works by acting upon tissue cells called mast cells, blocking their release of chemicals which produce the local inflammatory response to an allergy.

It's very important if you have a food allergy, even more so when you have one that produces violent reactions such as the peanut, that you check every ingredient in ready-made products you buy and, as much as it may seem a nuisance, you really do need to check restaurant menus carefully. Don't feel embarrassed to question catering staff closely on the contents of meals you may be about to eat.

Maggie, who has lactose intolerance, has found that using a product called Lactaid (containing the lactose enzyme) has helped her enormously. She describes it as a godsend because it means she can now have 'treated' milk in her diet. It's available in two forms, either a liquid enzyme or tablets. The liquid drops convert the lactose in any type of milk into digestible sugars before drinking. The tablets should be swallowed immediately before eating or drinking anything which may contain lactose.

For more information you can ring a Freephone helpline on 0800 581 342 Monday to Friday between 9 a.m. and 2 p.m.

My best tip for food allergy is to avoid strenuously foods known to contain the allergen to which you are particularly sensitive – especially when your reaction is frightening. This is obviously much easier if it is an item not regularly used in cooking.

Eczema and dermatitis

There are many products that can be prescribed for dry skin conditions, such as emollients to help moisturise the skin or steroids (taken topically or orally). Steroids are near-relatives of many of the natural hormones produced in our body. For instance, our adrenal glands secrete them when we're injured or under stress and these hormones are natural, cortisone-type healing and calming agents. Other steroids are secreted internally to control the body's reproductive functions.

The steroids taken – unofficially – by some sports people are called anabolic steroids and can cause a temporary increase in the mass and tone of the muscles of the body, as well as the speed with which the muscles work. These should not be confused with topical steroids used to treat dry skin conditions, reducing the redness and itchiness. They shouldn't be used on large areas of the body for a long time – say, daily for many weeks. Over-use of topical steroids, particularly the stronger ones, may make the skin so thin it can be easily damaged or allow the active ingredient to pass through and affect other parts of the body (especially on the face in infants and children, women who are pregnant, the elderly and people with kidney problems).

Topical steroids are particularly useful treatments in dry skin conditions such as eczema, dermatitis and psoriasis, helping to reduce redness, itchiness and dampen down any inflammation. These creams contain topical steroids such as hydrocortisone, betamethasone (Betnovate range), clobetasone butyrate (Eumovate Cream), beclomethasone dipropionate (Propaderm Cream), or clobetasol propionate (Dermovate range), for example. Sometimes infection can also be a problem in these skin conditions and where this is the case, a topical steroid cream with an antibacterial agent and/or an anti-fungal agent can be effective, for example a cream such as Dermovate-NN Ointment which contains clobetasol propionate (a topical steroid), neomycin (an antibacterial agent) and nystatin (an anti-candidal agent).

Evening Primrose Oil (Epogam) can be useful in .coping with eczema. Its major active constituent is gamolenic acid, also known as gamma-linolenic acid (GLA). It had been thought for some time that patients with atopic eczema may not be able to use dietary linoleic acid normally, and essential nutrient which, to perform its functions, must be converted within the body to GLA. Research carried out by Scotia Pharmaceuticals showed that eczema sufferers fail to convert linoleic acid to GLA normally and do not make enough GLA for normal skin structure and function. So adding GLA to the diet can help correct this biochemical abnormality.

It's worth remembering that once the eczema improves, the dosage may be reduced to a lower maintenance dose, but if treatment stops the patient's eczema may recur. According to the National Eczema Society, Epogam may take eight to twelve weeks before it is effective. The main benefit appears to be a reduction both of the itch and of the need for steroids and antibiotics. So far no major adverse effects have been reported although nausea, indigestion and headaches have occurred occasionally.

Sometimes your doctor may prescribe antihistamine tablets when itching really does become unbearable or uncontrollable.

You can combat the dryness, itching and flaking by preserving the moisture content of the skin. Avoid harsh or highly perfumed soaps or bath additives; instead, try using emollient soaps, creams and specially made bath oils, and when bathing use warm water instead of hot. Give your skin a good long soak so that it has a chance to absorb the emollients. (Moisturising bath oils can make the surface of the bath slippery, so do be careful about getting in and out.)

Examples of products you can buy over the counter include Cream E45, Diprobath, Emulsiderm Emollient, Oilatum Emollient, Polytar Emollient, Probase 3 Cream, Ultrabase, Unguentum Merck. Evening Primrose Oil may be soothing for dry skin conditions.

Keep your own or your child's skin away from direct contact with wool or other rough fabrics – choose soft, pure cotton instead. Keep fingernails short and use only gentle cleansing products. Contact the National Eczema Society for a list of cotton-goods stockists for adults and children alike.

If you suffer from contact dermatitis, protect your hands when using household cleansing fluids or chemicals, etc, and avoid contact with metals, dyes or even washing powders which may cause you problems. You can buy a range of household products, such as washing powder and fabric conditioner, which are designed for those with sensitive skin. Using a cream such as Savlon Barrier Cream can protect sensitive skin as it forms a barrier against potential irritants such as detergents and chemicals. Codella is another protective cream for working hands.

If you're not sure of the cause, consult your doctor, who may choose to carry out allergy tests. A mild hydrocortisone cream will ease discomfort by reducing inflammation and calming irritated skin. Hydrocortisone provides anti-inflammatory action yet is the least potent topical corticosteroid available.

Choose products which are hypo-allergenic (do not contain allergens such as perfumes, preservatives, lanolin, etc). Other products will be clearly marked perfume-free and some will even be preservative-free. Products containing alcohol, such as skin toners, aren't really suitable for anyone with eczema or a tendency to dry skin because alcohol can dry the skin. Baby products may not always be as gentle on the skin as you would think because they too can include perfumes and preservatives.

If you are going to use a product for the first time, particularly in the case of children's face-paints or depilatory creams to remove unwanted hair, it is wise to test a small area of skin first.

If you know what plays a contributory factor in your eczema then try to avoid it. Easier said than done, I know, in some cases. But if house dust could irritate your skin you can try to minimise the problem by taking steps outlined on pages 82–4.

Some sufferers find that their condition can be aggravated by heat, for instance by sitting in a centrally heated room. If you find that is true in your case, then it's wise to avoid any form of heat wherever you can, be it sunlight or even having a glass of alcohol, which opens up the blood vessels just under the skin and makes you feel hot.

Many sufferers have told me that they feel very guilty and self-conscious about scratching. The itch is often so bad they can't avoid attacking it. When skin is scratched so much that it bleeds, it can become vulnerable to infection, which in the long run only exacerbates pain and discomfort. The trick is to minimise the damage. Keep nails clean and short by filing daily – cutting leaves sharp edges. Older children and adults may find that gently rubbing or pressing the itchy area is a satisfactory alternative to scratching. Applying moisturiser when there's the urge to scratch will cool the skin, and reduce the damage caused by scratching. And no matter how young or old someone is, distraction is always more helpful than shouting 'Stop it!'

Urticaria

Fortunately, most cases of urticaria tend to resolve themselves in due course, and in the meantime antihistamine tablets prescribed by your doctor or recommended by your pharmacist usually relieve the symptoms and keep the condition under control. For mild cases, soothing creams containing antihistamine which stop the effects of histamine on the blood vessels beneath the skin, or creams and lotions containing calamine lotion help calm down any swelling and itching by cooling the skin, especially if these preparations contain menthol, phenol or camphor.

If angio-oedema is severe and breathing becomes difficult, emergency treatment by injection may be necessary to reduce the swelling.

Common sense prevails when dealing with urticaria. If you know certain foods trigger urticaria try to avoid them wherever you can. The common ones are shellfish and strawberries, nuts and some fruits, and drugs such as penicillin or aspirin. Having said that, there are many people who never discover what causes them to develop a rash. If this happens to you, you could try jotting down the things you've eaten, or substances you've come into contact with, to see whether that will provide a clue.

For those whose allergies can be overwhelming and even life-threatening, emergency treatment should be carried at all times. An adrenaline injection or inhaler can be prescribed by your doctor. You could also wear a disc from MedicAlert (071 833 3034) around your neck to warn of an allergy.

There is hope for the future. According to the British Allergy Foundation there are new drugs in the pipeline which, it is believed, will totally change the way allergies are treated in the next century. Called cytokines, they are chemicals which are involved in controlling the development of histamine-releasing cells (mast cells) and white blood cells. Assuming all the safety checks are successful, these drugs hold great promise for the future.

Other research involves the ways in which the allergic pathways – reactions in the body that result in an allergic reaction – can be interrupted.

So, don't get too excited yet, but watch this space. The whole field is quite exciting when one considers the not-too-distant possibilities.

DESENSITISATION

What other steps can you take to cope? Well, there are three main ways of dealing with an allergy: avoidance of, or reduced contact with, the allergen; drugs, in particular steroids or antihistamines as we've discussed earlier; and desensitisation. The latter treatment offers protection against the allergens you are already allergic to and, it is claimed, for those that you *could* become allergic to. Together with most doctors, I'm sceptical about desensitisation treatments, especially those which claim to protect you against reactions that have yet to occur. Some clinics offer neutralisation therapy which involves small doses of allergens being injected with the aim of the body building up a tolerance. But I remain doubtful.

Perhaps the best way to cope is avoidance, if you are fortunate enough to be able to trace what triggers your allergy. Experts believe that it's better to get to the root of the problem by minimising contact with an allergen rather than just relying on drug management. Of course, with something like hay fever it's virtually impossible to avoid pollen totally – unless you can afford to move house and live by the sea, which few of us can!

If you don't know what triggers your allergy you can try to keep a diary of symptoms, which is how many migraine sufferers pinpoint what triggers their attacks. You'll need to record what your symptoms are each day, what the weather was like, what you might have eaten and who or what you came into contact with. You may notice a pattern of behaviour forming which will help to pinpoint your trigger factors. This method is worth a go because you really have nothing to lose, and there'll be no unwanted side-effects.

SKIN TESTING

Skin testing may be able to help you identify an allergen. Prick tests involve small and weak droplets containing common allergens being applied to the skin. If a reaction occurs, such as weals or a red patch, then it's likely that you are allergic to that particular allergen. However, many doctors don't rely on the skin prick test alone to identify an allergen, as it's not always completely effective.

DIET

I do feel it's important that anyone thinking of undergoing an elimination diet to try to find out which foods may trigger an allergy should do so only under the medical supervision of a doctor or a dietician as they can give proper advice and correct nutritional information. This is particularly important when it comes to tampering with a child's diet.

COMPLEMENTARY TREATMENTS

My thoughts on this are that if you have tried the conventional, traditional approach and your symptoms have not been relieved, then why not try an alternative therapy, provided you go to a practitioner who is approved by their professional organisation, if there is one. (If there isn't, then it's not advisable.) Also, make sure that they're insured against negligence and that you can afford their fees, since you'll have to pay in most cases. And don't go if your doctor has advised against it.

Most practitioners of unconventional therapies prefer the use of the term 'complementary' medicine rather than 'alternative' because they feel their treatment should work side by side with more conventional methods. I'm in favour of their treatments in certain cases, but do let your doctor and the complementary practitioner know that you're seeking the help of them both. And listen to their advice and their opinions on the value or the dangers.

Acupuncture

Acupuncture has been an accepted form of treatment in China for around 5000 years and these days more and more people in the West are turning to it. Many people believe it is extremely effective in easing a wide variety of conditions by – in simple terms – stimulating the patient's own healing responses.

Acupuncture aims to correct any disharmony within the body – to achieve a balance between Yin and Yang. An imbalance, they say, can lead to disease. There are different traditions of acupuncture but they all revolve around the basic principle that the body has an intricate network of linking pathways, 'meridians', which carry our vital 'energies' through the body. These cannot be seen but can be detected using special techniques and can be likened, though loosely, to the nerve pathways known to Western doctors.

During acupuncture very fine needles are inserted into several 'acupoints' according to the problem being treated. By inserting needles or by using pressure, the correct flow and balance of energies can be restored. One theory is that acupuncture stimulates the brain to produce endorphins, the body's natural painkillers.

The National Asthma Campaign has pointed out, however, that some trials have shown that acupuncture can relax and might protect against exercise-induced asthma, but that it doesn't seem to be particularly helpful in the long-term management of the condition. As for hypnosis and relaxation, techniques such as yoga could be of benefit by helping to relieve stress.

Homoeopathy

Homoeopathy is a system which works on the theory that less is more and that like cures like. Symptoms are treated by giving a minute dose of a substance which, if given in larger quantities to a healthy person, would actually cause those symptoms. Even in conventional medicine this principle is sometimes used – for instance, controlled doses of radiation are given to cure cancer which can be *caused* by too much radiation. No one has so far been able to explain exactly how it works, however, as it does not conform to our accepted knowledge of scientific medicine, though one theory is that a form of radiation energy is released which stimulates the body's own healing mechanisms. Homoeopaths point out that we don't understand how many modern drugs work, but we do know that a few have unpleasant side-effects.

Osteopathy

Osteopathy is the most orthodox of the unorthodox therapies which believes that many diseases are due to parts of the skeleton being misplaced and should consequently be treated by gentle methods of adjustment. Osteopaths use a variety of techniques ranging from gentle massage or stretching movements to manipulation.

Eczema sufferers have found that alternative treatments such as homoeopathy, herbalism (particularly Chinese herbal medicine) and osteopathy have helped relieve symptoms. Remember, though, that eczema has no specific cure and that atopic eczema can suddenly clear up on its own and can return just as unexpectedly.

Finally a word of advice if you are considering trying alternative therapies. Do consult your doctor and, especially in the case of asthma, you do still need to carry on with your preventative treatments, as well as the medicines you use to relieve an asthma attack.

HELPFUL ADDRESSES

UNITED KINGDOM

Action Against Allergy, 24–26 High Street, Hampton Hill, Middlesex TW12 1PD.
Members can receive a newsletter, suppliers list – quick reference sources on the supply of additive-free, natural and organic foods, non-allergenic products, fabrics and bedding, household cleaners, cosmetics etc – as well as information packs. The charity also holds a reference list of experts – some private, some NHS, some both – and can inform people of their nearest likely specialist. Please contact the society by post with an SAE.

The British Allergy Foundation, St Bartholomew's Hospital, West Smithfield, London EC1A 7BE. Tel: 071 600 6127.
Set up in 1991, the British Allergy Foundation is the first national charity concerned with every type of allergy, including hay fever, asthma, perennial rhinitis, childhood eczema, nettle rash and food allergy. Its aims are to increase the awareness and understanding of allergy as well as providing funds for research projects.

The Department of the Environment's Pollution Helpline. Tel: 0800 556677 (calls are free).
For information on air pollution levels across the country, health ideas and ideas on how you can reduce pollution.

The Holiday Care Service, 2 Old Bank Chambers, Station Road, Horley, Surrey RH6 9HW. Tel: 0293 774535.
Provides information about holidays for those with disabilities, such as asthma.

National Asthma Campaign, Providence House, Providence Place, London N1 0NT. Tel: 071 226 2260. Asthma Helpline 0345 01 02 03 (calls charged at local rates).
The helpline is staffed by trained asthma nurses and offers advice and counselling to asthma sufferers and their carers. It is open weekdays from 1–9 p.m. The campaigns aims are to fund research, build awareness about asthma and how it is treated and to offer support to people with the condition. Its quarterly newspaper explains scientific discoveries and new treatments. Its local branches provide personal and practical support for sufferers.

National Eczema Society, 4 Tavistock Place, London WC1H 9RA. Tel: 071 388 4097.
The society was set up to support, educate, inform and to raise money for research. For details of the society's wide range of literature, including the quarterly journal *Exchange*, and for information on membership, send a large SAE.

Peanut Allergy – if you or a member of your family is allergic to peanuts you may be interested to know that David Reading, whose daughter Sarah died after eating a lemon meringue pie containing peanuts, has launched a national campaign to tighten food labelling law. The campaign is also to gather information which could prove life-saving, for example lists of safe and unsafe products as well as forming a national registers of sufferers. You can write to him, sending an SAE, at Wey Close, Ash, Aldershot, Hampshire GU12 6LY.

The Pollen Research Unit, University of North London, 166–220 Holloway Road, London N7 8DB. For advice on pollens write including an SAE.

AUSTRALIA

Eczema/Dermatitis Association of South Australia, PO Box 331, St Marys 5042.

The National Asthma Campaign, PO Box 360, Woden, ACT 2606, Australia. Tel: 06 282 3265.

CANADA

Association Pulmonaire de Quebec, 3440 Avenue de l'Hotel de Ville, Montreal, Quebec H2X 3B4, Canada. Tel: 514 845 3129.

The Lung Association, National Office, 1900 City Park Drive, Suite 508, Gloucester ONK1 J1A3.

Parents of Allergic and Asthmatic Children, Box No 4500, Edmonton, Alberta TEE 6K2.

INDEX

Lot No Wed.

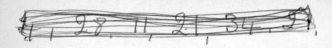

(16)

4 . 11 . 21 . 27 . 28 . 34 ,